PERGAMON GENERAL PSYCHOLOGY SERIES

Editors: Arnold P. Goldstein, *Syracuse University*
Leonard Krasner, *SUNY, Stony Brook*

Hypnosis, Imagination, and Human Potentialities

PGPS-46

Hypnosis, Imagination, and Human Potentialities

THEODORE X. BARBER,
NICHOLAS P. SPANOS,
and JOHN F. CHAVES

Medfield Foundation and State Hospital
Medfield, Massachusetts

PERGAMON PRESS INC.

New York · Toronto · Oxford · Sydney

PERGAMON PRESS INC.
Maxwell House, Fairview Park, Elmsford, N.Y. 10523

PERGAMON OF CANADA LTD.
207 Queen's Quay West, Toronto 117, Ontario

PERGAMON PRESS LTD.
Headington Hill Hall, Oxford

PERGAMON PRESS (AUST.) PTY. LTD.
Rushcutters Bay, Sydney, N.S.W.

Library of Congress Cataloging in Publication Data

Barber, Theodore Xenophon, 1927-
   Hypnosis, imagination, and human potentialities.

   (Pergamon general psychology series, 46)
     1. Hypnotism—Therapeutic use.   I. Spanos, Nicholas
P., joint author. II. Chaves, John F., joint author.
III. T Title. [DNLM: 1. Hypnosis. BF1141 B234h 1974]
RC495.B34   1974   615'.8512   73-19539
ISBN 0-08-017932-0
ISBN 0-08-017931-2 (pbk.)

Printed in the United States of America

Contents

The Authors...

Theodore X. Barber (Ph.D., American University) is Chief Psychologist at the State Hospital in Medfield, Massachusetts and Director of Psychological Research at the Medfield Foundation. He has published 130 scientific papers on hypnosis and related topics and three previous books (*Hypnosis: A Scientific Approach; LSD, Marihuana, Yoga and Hypnosis;* and *Biofeedback and Self-Control*). He is President of the Massachusetts Psychological Association and has served as President of the Hypnosis Division of the American Psychological Association.

Nicholas P. Spanos (Ph.D., Boston University) is Senior Research Scientist at the Medfield Foundation, and Clinical Consultant to the Day Care Program at Medfield State Hospital. His clinical activities include group, family, and individual psychotherapy, and his research publications have been in the areas of imagination, hypnosis, and behavior modification.

John F. Chaves (Ph.D., Northeastern University) is Senior Research Psychologist at the Medfield Foundation and Lecturer in Psychology at Northeastern University. His publications have been in the areas of sensory and perceptual processes, hypnosis, and social influence. He also has a professional interest in rehabilitation and developmental disabilities.

Preface

In this book, we criticize the traditional explanation of hypnotism and we present an alternative explanation. The traditional explanation pivots around the concept of "hypnosis" or "hypnotic trance" and is based on assumptions such as the following (Barber, 1972):

1. There exists a state of consciousness that is fundamentally different from the waking state and the deep sleep state. This distinct state is labeled "hypnosis," "the hypnotic state," or "trance."
2. Hypnosis may occasionally occur spontaneously, but it is usually induced by certain kinds of procedures that are labeled "hypnotic inductions" or "trance inductions."
3. Hypnosis is not a momentary condition that lasts only for a few seconds. On the contrary, when a person has been placed in a hypnotic state, he remains in it for a period of time and he is typically brought out of it by a command from the hypnotist, such as "Wake up!"
4. There are levels or depths of hypnosis; that is, hypnosis can vary from light to medium to very deep.
5. As the person goes deeper into hypnosis, he becomes increasingly responsive to a wide variety of suggestions, including suggestions for anesthesia, age regression, hallucination, and amnesia.

We do not accept any of the above five assumptions. In this book, we shall criticize these assumptions, which underlie the "hypnotic trance" viewpoint, and we shall present another way of understanding hypnotism. We shall argue that concepts such as "hypnosis," "hypnotic trance," and "depth of hypnosis" are unnecessary and misleading, and that subjects respond to suggestions and experience the phenomena associated with the word "hypnotism" to the extent that (a) they have positive attitudes, motivations, and expectancies toward the test situation and, consequently, (b) they allow themselves to think and imagine with the themes that are suggested. We shall also show how our viewpoint broadens conceptions of human capabilities or potentialities and how it suggests new lines of interesting research.

Specifically, in this book, we shall extend our earlier work on hypnotism (Barber, 1961a, 1967, 1969b, 1970; Chaves, 1968; Spanos, 1970) by further examining "hypnotic" phenomena and the factors that are present when a subject is said to be "hypnotized." The present text grows out of our earlier work in two ways:

1. In our previous work, we looked closely at a variety of phenomena that have been historically associated with hypnotism. These phenomena included age regression, hallucinations, amnesia, time distortion, heightened learning proficiency, posthypnotic behavior, and physiological alterations such as formation of "blisters." We showed that these and other phenomena have been commonly viewed in a very misleading way and that they are basically different from what they have been assumed to be. In the present text, we extend our previous endeavors by showing that additional phenomena—for instance, stage hypnotism and "painless surgery" produced by hypnotism—have also been traditionally misunderstood.

2. Our previous research also showed that many situational factors play a role in determining whether subjects manifest "hypnotic" behaviors. These factors include, for example, the manner in which the situation is defined to the subject, the wording or phrasing of the suggestions, and the tone of voice in which the suggestions are administered. The situational variables, however, do not directly affect the subjects' performance. Instead, they affect performance indirectly by first influencing a set of mediating variables that include the subjects' attitudes, motivations, and expectancies and their readiness to think and imagine with the themes that are suggested. In the present text, we move forward by looking closely at the latter set of variables that mediate performance in hypnotic situations.

A satisfactory understanding of hypnotism will be attained only when we are able to specify clearly the relevant antecedent variables, the variables that mediate between the antecedent variables and the subject's performance, and the precise nature of the experiences and behaviors that are elicited in the situation. We believe that some important antecedent variables have been specified in our previous work and that important mediating variables are more clearly formulated in the present text. Also, we believe that, as work continues in this area, additional factors and additional interactions among complex factors will be more clearly formulated and a broader understanding of hypnotism will be attained.

Since this book presents a viewpoint toward hypnotism and has its own particular story to tell, it does not attempt to cover the vast literature that derives from the "hypnotic trance" viewpoint. For an overview of alternative conceptualizations, the reader is urged to consult Conn and Conn (1967), Estabrooks (1943), Fromm and Shor (1972), Hilgard (1965), Moss (1965), and Shor and Orne (1965). Also, this book does not attempt to cover the applications of "hypnosis" in psychotherapy. Readers interested in psychotherapy should read such texts as Erickson (1967), Gill and Brenman (1959), Schneck (1965), Watkins (1949), and Wolberg (1948, 1972).

T. X. Barber wrote the original drafts of Chapters 1-7, 9, and 10; N. P. Spanos wrote the first draft of Chapter 11; and J. F. Chaves wrote the original versions of Chapter 8 and Appendix B. Each of the co-authors then worked at revising all of the chapters and appendices. Writing of the book was made possible by two research grants (MH-19152 and MH-21294) from the National Institute of Mental Health, U. S. Public Health Service. We are deeply indebted to the National Institute of Mental Health for the continuous financial support of our research. We are also indebted to C. Richard Chapman who critically read Chapter 8 and Appendix B, and to the following who critically read the entire manuscript: Shirley Aleo, Frederic Altaffer, Doris Steele Brown, Wilfried De Moor, Ambellur Frederick, Carol Goldman, Martin W. Ham, Richard F. Q. Johnson, Roberta Kaplan, John D. McPeake, William Meeker, Janice Parker, Joanne Rubino, Barbara Slack, Monte Stavis, Lisa Tulin, and Priscilla C. Walker.

T.X.B.
N.P.S.
J.F.C.

PART A

Introduction and Analogies

CHAPTER 1

Introduction

This book has two major purposes. First, it presents a conception of hypnotism that differs in many respects from the way it has been commonly conceived. Second, it tries to show how the new conception broadens our understanding of human capabilities and potentialities. Since this book is about "hypnotism," let us first clarify this term by describing the phenomena that are usually associated with it.

Typically, one person (the hypnotist) administers a hypnotic induction procedure to another person (the subject). For example, the hypnotist may ask the subject to stare at a blinking light and then may give repeated suggestions for eye-heaviness and eye-closure: "Your eyes are becoming tired and heavy . . . heavier and heavier. . . . Your lids are as heavy as lead . . . so heavy. . . . The strain on your eyes is becoming greater and greater. . . ." If the subject has not closed his eyes by this time, the hypnotist may state directly: "Close your eyes now." The hypnotist then continues with repeated suggestions of relaxation, drowsiness, sleep, and suggestions that the subject is entering a hypnotic state: "Your muscles are relaxing . . . more and more relaxed. . . . Comfortable and relaxed, breathing regularly and deeply, thinking of nothing. . . . Drowsy and sleepy. . . . More and more drowsy and sleepy . . . a deep, comfortable, restful sleep. . . . In a deep hypnotic state. . . ." When hypnotism is being used for experimental purposes, the hypnotic induction procedure usually continues for about 10 to 15 minutes.

When exposed to these repeated suggestions of eye-closure, relaxation, drowsiness, sleep, and hypnosis, some subjects show *a "hypnotic" appearance*, that is, they appear very relaxed, drowsy, sleepy, or lethargic, and they may talk slowly and may seem to lack spontaneity and initiative. Also, some of the

3

subjects who have been exposed to the hypnotic induction procedure *are very responsive to tests of suggestibility*. For instance, the hypnotist may tell the subject, "Your right arm is rigid . . . solid . . . a piece of steel . . . you cannot bend it." The subject may not bend his arm even though he tries to do so. Next, the hypnotist may tell the subject repeatedly that his hand is dull, numb, and insensitive—it has lost all feelings and sensations. He then moves the flame of a match across the subject's palm and the subject seems to be insensitive to it. The hypnotist may then give a test suggestion for age regression: "Time is going backwards. . . . It is 1940. . . . You are six years of age. . . . You are in the first grade in school." The subject may state that he is six years old. When asked to write his name, he may print it in large letters and the writing may resemble that of a child in the first grade. Many other types of test suggestions may also be given before the end of the hypnotic session. These may include suggestions for arm levitation ("Your arm is becoming light and is rising in the air"), visual hallucination ("Open your eyes and see a cat on your lap"), and amnesia ("You will forget everything that occurred"). After the subject is told to awaken, he may state *that he felt he was hypnotized*. In addition, *he may report changes in body feelings*—for example, that he felt as if he were floating or as if his body were separated from his mind.

Briefly stated, when we use the term "hypnotism," we are thinking of a situation in which the hypnotist's suggestions influence the subject (a) to appear relaxed, drowsy, and lethargic (that is, to show a *"hypnotic" appearance*), (b) to manifest a *high level of responsiveness to test suggestions* for limb rigidity, hand insensitivity or anesthesia, age regression, etc., (c) to *report changes in body feelings*, and (d) to *report that he was hypnotized*. It is the task of behavioral scientists to explain how and why these four sets of phenomena occur. More specifically, the scientist must attempt to answer questions such as the following: When exposed to a hypnotic induction procedure, why do some individuals appear relaxed, drowsy, sleepy, or lethargic while others do not show this "hypnotic" appearance? Which factors in the hypnotic induction procedure are effective and which are irrelevant in producing a high level of response to test suggestions? Why do some subjects but not others report changes in body feelings or report that they were hypnotized? We shall attempt to answer these and many related questions in this book.

During the past century, many attempts have been made to explain the "hypnotic" experiences and behaviors that were described above. These endeavors have given rise to two major viewpoints. One viewpoint attempts to explain the experiences and behaviors by postulating (a) that hypnotic induction procedures give rise to a special state and (b) that the special state (hypnotic trance) gives rise to a "hypnotic" appearance, a high level of responsiveness to test suggestions, changes in body feelings, and reports of having been hypnotized. This orientation, which we shall label the *"hypnotic trance" viewpoint*, has been widely accepted. In fact, most people take it for granted that subjects who have been exposed to a hypnotic induction procedure manifest a "hypnotic" appearance, are responsive to test suggestions, report changes in body feelings, and report that they are hypnotized because they are in a special state—"hypnotic trance".

An alternative point of view, which is elaborated in the present text, might be labeled the *cognitive-behavioral viewpoint*. This approach proceeds to account for so-called "hypnotic" experiences and behaviors without postulating that the subjects are in a special state of "hypnotic trance." In fact, from the cognitive-behavioral viewpoint, the concept of *hypnotic trance* and related concepts—*hypnotized, hypnosis*, and *hypnotic state*—are not only unnecessary but also misleading in explaining the phenomena. From the cognitive-behavioral viewpoint, *subjects carry out so-called "hypnotic" behaviors when they have positive attitudes, motivations, and expectations toward the test situation which lead to a willingness to think and imagine with the themes that are suggested.* We shall develop and amplify this theoretical viewpoint in this text.[1] Let us begin by providing a short overview of the chapters that follow.

OVERVIEW OF CHAPTERS 2-11

In Chapter 2, three analogies will be used to highlight the differences between the traditional "hypnotic trance" viewpoint and our own cognitive-behavioral approach. Traditionally, the responsive subject in a hypnotic situation has been thought to resemble the sleepwalker. We shall present data indicating that this analogy is misleading—the responsive hypnotic subject differs in every important respect from the sleepwalker. We shall present a different analogy, which sees the good hypnotic subject as resembling the person who is reading a novel or is observing a motion picture. The responsive hypnotic subject, and also the reader of a novel and the observer of a motion picture, has intense and vivid experiences that are produced by the words or communications he is receiving (from the hypnotist, the book, or the screen).

Chapters 3 and 4 pertain to the art of "hypnotizing." Here we explain how skilled hypnotists administer hypnotic induction procedures in order to produce positive attitudes, motivations, and expectancies toward the test situation and to lead the subject to think and imagine with the themes that are suggested. When the various factors in the hypnotic induction procedure have led the subject to think and imagine with the themes that are suggested, the subject will tend to manifest a high level of responsiveness to test suggestions (Chapter 3), to show a "hypnotic" appearance, to report changes in body feelings, and to report that he was hypnotized (Chapter 4).

The theory of "hypnotic" behavior that we present in this text emphasizes the importance of the subject's attitudes, motivations, and expectancies and the critical role of thinking and imagining with the themes that are suggested. Research that indicates the importance of these factors is summarized in Chapters 5 and 6.

In Chapters 7, 8, and 9, we critically reevaluate a series of seemingly extraordinary "hypnotic" phenomena. The first part of this section (Chapter 7) discusses several "amazing" phenomena that have been associated with hypnotism, such as the production of perceptual and physiological alterations, age regression, visual hallucinations, and unusual cognitive processes. In Chapter 8, we explain how hypnotism and suggestions are used to perform surgical operations. In the last chapter in this section (Chapter 9), a series of factors are specified, about which very few individuals seem to know, that explain the "marvelous" events of stage hypnotism.

In Chapter 10, we show how our viewpoint gives rise to a broadened conception of human capabilities or potentialities. Also, at the end of this chapter, we outline methods that can be used to teach individuals to tolerate pain, to respond to a variety of suggestions, and to experience a series of interesting or useful phenomena that have been traditionally associated with hypnotism.

In the final chapter (Chapter 11), we ask: Where do we go from here? The limitations of our formulation are stated and a series of investigations are proposed that can enhance our understanding of hypnotism.

SUMMARY

It has been traditionally assumed that subjects manifest "hypnotic" behaviors when they are in a special state—"hypnotic trance." In this book, we present a cognitive-behavioral theory that challenges the traditional viewpoint. Our theory views concepts such as *hypnotized, hypnosis, hypnotic state,* and *hypnotic trance* as misleading—as not helpful in explaining the behaviors historically associated with hypnotism. From our viewpoint, subjects carry out "hypnotic" behaviors when they have positive attitudes, motivations, and expectancies toward the test situation and, consequently, when they are willing to think and imagine with the themes that are suggested.

NOTES

[1] In many respects, our theory of hypnotism is in agreement with the theory presented by Sarbin and his associates. However, the two theories differ primarily in that Sarbin's is based on the social-psychological concept of "role" while ours does not utilize this concept. Sarbin's theory has been presented in detail in a recent important book (Sarbin & Coe, 1972), and it will be discussed in Chapters 6 and 11 of the present text.

CHAPTER 2

Analogies

THE SLEEPWALKER AND THE HYPNOTIC SUBJECT

Traditionally, the "good" subject in a hypnotic situation has been thought to resemble the sleepwalker. As Hilgard (1969a) pointed out, "Hypnosis is commonly considered to be a 'state' perhaps resembling the state in which the sleepwalker finds himself, hence the term 'somnambulist' as applied to the deeply hypnotized person." This notion is a very old one, stretching back to the early nineteenth century when "hypnotic trance" was thought to be a condition resembling sleep. It has influenced contemporary ideas about hypnotism in a number of important ways. One example is the fact that hypnotic induction procedures typically instruct the subject to become drowsy and to go into a deep sleep. Let us evaluate this analogy by first looking carefully at the sleepwalker and then at the responsive subject in a hypnotic experiment.

A number of recent studies (Jacobson, Kales, Lehmann, & Zweizig, 1965; Kales, Jacobson, Paulson, Kales, & Walter, 1966; Pai, 1946) indicate that the sleepwalker manifests four sets of characteristics:

First, when the sleepwalker arises from his bed at night, the electroencephalogram (EEG) shows that he is sleeping (stage 3 or 4 of sleep) and, when the sleepwalking episode is brief, the EEG shows that he remains asleep.

Second, the sleepwalker shows rigid or shuffling movements, a drastically reduced awareness of his surroundings, a low level of motor skill, and a blank stare. He rarely replies when someone speaks to him. To get his attention, it is usually necessary to continue talking to him or to interrupt his movements. When the sleepwalker does reply, he tends to mumble or to speak in a vague or detached manner.

Third, when the sleepwalker is told to wake up, he does not awaken. Persistent measures are needed to awaken him. For example, it may be necessary to shake him or to repeat his name over and over, each time more loudly.

Finally, when the sleepwalker is awakened in the morning, or if he is awakened during his sleepwalking, he shows no indication of remembering the episode.

Subjects who are said to be "hypnotized" are often termed *somnambulists* or *somnambules* with the clear implication that they resemble the sleepwalker. Laymen commonly believe that subjects exposed to hypnotic induction procedures resemble the sleepwalker in that they are "half asleep," have a low level of awareness, are detached from their surroundings, and show amnesia on awakening. This belief is fallacious. Knowledgeable workers in this area agree that the so-called "hypnotized" subject differs from the sleepwalker in every important respect.

First, the EEG of the "hypnotized" subject does not remotely resemble the EEG of the sleepwalker. Judging from EEG criteria, the sleepwalker is asleep, whereas the subject who is said to be "hypnotized" is awake. More specifically, "hypnotized" subjects do not show changes on the EEG that might clearly distinguish them from subjects who are said to be "awake." The EEG of the so-called "hypnotized" subject changes continually, in the same way as in any "normally awake" person, with whatever instructions or suggestions he is given or with whatever activities he is carrying out (Barber, 1961c; Chertok & Kramarz, 1959).[1]

Second, in the "hypnotized" subject, but *not* in the sleepwalker, characteristics such as a blank stare, a rigid facial expression, and an unwillingness to talk have been produced by suggestions to become relaxed, drowsy, and sleepy, and they can be easily removed by suggestions—for example, by suggestions to be alert.

Third, although the sleepwalker does not awaken when he is simply told to do so, practically all subjects who are said to be "hypnotized" open their eyes and "awaken" when they are simply told, "The experiment is over" or "Wake up."[2]

Finally, although sleepwalkers do not remember their sleepwalking, *no* hypnotic subject has ever forgotten the events occurring during the hypnotic session when he was told during the session that he should remember what occurred (Barber, 1962b; Orne, 1966; Watkins, 1966). Furthermore, practically all "hypnotized" subjects state postexperimentally that they remember what occurred if suggestions for amnesia are not given during the hypnotic session (Barber & Calverley, 1966b; Hilgard, 1966).[3]

In brief, the traditional analogy that compared the "hypnotized" subject to the sleepwalker is misleading. The subject who is responding to suggestions in a hypnotic situation does not resemble the sleepwalker. Instead, he more closely resembles the person who is reading an interesting novel or is observing an interesting motion picture. Let us now turn to the latter two analogies.

TWO CLARIFYING ANALOGIES

The processes involved in responding to test suggestions—for example, suggestions for limb rigidity, anesthesia, age regression, amnesia, etc.—are similar to those present when a person is reading an interesting novel or observing an interesting motion picture. When reading an interesting novel, a person thinks and imagines with the communications from the printed page. To the extent that he becomes engrossed or involved in his imaginings, he does not have contradictory thoughts such as "This is only a novel" or "This is only make-believe." Instead, he experiences a variety of emotions while empathizing and "living with" the characters. At times he experiences sadness and tears may cover his face. At times he may smile to himself and may laugh aloud. Along similar lines, Shor (1970) has pointed out that, when reading a novel, some individuals "think the thoughts in the story and they feel the emotions." Shor labeled this behavior the *book reading fantasy* and noted the following relevant characteristics:

> ... the reader creates the fantasy for his own purposes, to satisfy his own motives. The fantasy is not implanted in the mind by the words in the book. The reader is not forced to create the fantasy by the inexorable "suggestive" power of the words. The words do not express themselves with the reader's will held in abeyance. The reader is not too much asleep to control his own mind. He is not an automaton obeying the commands of his master. The words in the book have no ideomotor powers in their own right except insofar as the reader deliberately gives them expression. The reader is deliberately using the words in the book for his own ends [p. 93].

In brief, we believe that the person who is responding to suggestions in a hypnotic situation resembles the person who is thinking and imagining with the words of a novel. The concept of "hypnotic trance" is no more helpful in explaining the experiences of the hypnotic subject than in explaining the experiences of the reader. From our viewpoint, it is just as misleading to "explain" the experiences of the hypnotic subject by saying that he is in a "hypnotic trance" as it is to "explain" the experiences of the book-reader by saying that he is in a "hypnotic trance."

The processes involved in responding to suggestions in a hypnotic situation also resemble those present when a person has a variety of emotional experiences while observing a motion picture. At a movie, the person thinks with the communications from the screen. As he becomes engrossed or involved in the action, he does not have negative thoughts such as "These are only actors," "This is just a story that someone made up," or "This is just a series of lights playing upon a screen." Since he thinks and imagines with the communications, he feels, emotes, and experiences in line with the intentions of the writer of the screenplay—he may feel happy or sad and may empathize, laugh, weep, experience horror or shock, etc. It is misleading to claim that he is having intense experiences and emotions as he observes the motion picture because he has entered a special state—"hypnotic trance." He is having intense experiences while observing the movie because he is thinking and imagining with the communications from the screen.

In a similar way, when a person is responding to suggestions in a hypnotic situation, he is thinking and imagining with the communications that he is receiving. However, the person observing a motion picture and the person in a hypnotic situation are exposed to different kinds of communications. The communications from the movie are intended to elicit certain kinds of thoughts, emotions, and experiences—to feel excited or shocked, to empathize, to laugh or to cry, to feel happy or sad. The communications from the hypnotist are intended to elicit different types of thoughts, emotions, and experiences—to feel that an arm is light and is rising, to experience oneself as a child, to imagine vividly (or hallucinate), etc. When a person is receiving suggestions in a hypnotic situation, he has somewhat different experiences than when he is observing a motion picture, *not because he is in a different "state"* ("hypnotic trance") but because he is receiving different communications.

It should also be noted that a person who is observing a motion picture may have negative attitudes, motivations, and expectancies toward the performance and may fail to experience the emotions that the actors are attempting to communicate. He may be attending the movie unwillingly. He may have had a difficult and tiring day at the office, may have wanted to go to bed early in the evening, and may have come to the performance unwillingly in order to avoid an argument with his wife. He may not especially desire and may not expect to feel happy, sad, shocked, excited, or empathic. Given these kinds of attitudes, motivations, and expectancies, he may say to himself that this is just a movie and he is just watching actors perform their roles; he may remain continually aware that he is in an audience and that he is observing a deliberately contrived performance. Since he observes the movie in this uninvolved and distant manner, he does not think and imagine with the communications and he does not laugh, feel sad, empathize, or, more generally, feel, emote, and experience in line with the communications from the screen. We believe that this person resembles the subject who is unresponsive to suggestions in a hypnotic situation. Both individuals have negative attitudes, motivations, or expectancies toward the situation which prevent them from thinking and imagining with the communications they receive.

SUMMARY

Traditionally, the "hypnotized" subject has been thought to resemble the sleepwalker. This analogy is misleading. Instead, the processes involved in responding to suggestions in a hypnotic situation resemble those found when a person is experiencing sadness, happiness, empathy, excitement, shock, and a variety of other emotions as he reads an interesting novel or observes a motion picture. In each of these instances—when responding to suggestions in a hypnotic situation, when reading a novel, or when observing a movie—the person who has positive attitudes, motivations, and expectancies toward the situation thinks and imagines with the communications he is receiving.

NOTES

[1] Other physiological measures also vary in "hypnotized" subjects in the same way as in control subjects who are said to be "awake." Depending on the instructions or suggestions that the subject receives, both the "hypnotized" subject and the "waking control" subject at times show high levels and at times medium or low levels of heart rate, blood pressure, skin resistance, basal metabolic rate, respiration, peripheral blood flow, blood clotting time, oral temperature, and so forth (Barber, 1961c, 1970; Crasilneck & Hall, 1959; Levitt & Brady, 1963; Sarbin, 1956; Sarbin & Slagle, 1972; Timney & Barber, 1969). Furthermore, when specific types of suggestions (for example, suggestions of analgesia) produce physiological changes in subjects who are said to be "hypnotized," the suggestions also produce very similar physiological changes in control subjects who are said to be "awake" (Barber, 1961c, 1965b). For instance, in both "hypnotized" subjects and in control subjects, suggestions of analgesia or anesthesia at times reduce respiratory and electromyographic responses to noxious stimulation (Barber & Hahn, 1962).

[2] In very rare cases, a "hypnotized" subject does not open his eyes when told that the experiment is over. These rare cases are due to such reasons as the following: The subject may have actually fallen asleep, or he may not have fallen asleep but he (a) wants to remain a little longer in a relaxed or passive condition, (b) has been given a posthypnotic suggestion that he does not want to carry out, (c) is purposely resisting the hypnotist, (d) is testing the hypnotist's ability to control him, (e) is manifesting spite toward the hypnotist, or (f) is attempting to frighten the hypnotist by refusing to "awaken" (Weitzenhoffer, 1957, pp. 226-229; Williams, 1953).

[3] In rare instances, "hypnotized" subjects who are *not* given suggestions for amnesia state postexperimentally that they do not remember what occurred during the session. There are several reasons for viewing this apparent amnesia not as a spontaneous occurrence but as due to explicit or implicit suggestions: (a) In many of these cases, the subject had received suggestions for amnesia in a previous hypnotic session and may have generalized the suggestions for amnesia to apply to subsequent sessions as well. (b) Suggestions to sleep were administered during the hypnotic session. Since sleep is followed by amnesia, the suggestions to sleep included the implicit suggestion that the subject is expected to show amnesia on "awakening." (c) A substantial proportion of present-day subjects believe that "hypnotized" persons manifest amnesia (London, 1961) and that they will be considered "poor" subjects, the experimenter will be disappointed, and the experiment may be "spoiled" if they state postexperimentally that they remember what occurred.

* * *

Shor extract is from Shor, R.E. The three-factor theory of hypnosis as applied to the book-reading fantasy and to the concept of suggestion. Quoted from the October 1970 *International Journal of Clinical and Experimental Hypnosis*. Copyrighted by the Society for Clinical and Experimental Hypnosis, October, 1970.

PART B

The Art of "Hypnotizing"

CHAPTER 3

Enhancing Response to Suggestions

In experimental settings, "hypnotic induction procedures" typically consist of a series of standardized suggestions emphasizing relaxation, drowsiness, and sleep. These kinds of "hypnotic induction procedures" which are administered in the same way to all subjects, usually give rise to a relatively high level of responsiveness to test suggestions for arm levitation, limb rigidity, total body rigidity, sensory hallucination, amnesia, and posthypnotic behavior (Barber, 1969b). It is commonly assumed that the "hypnotic induction procedure" is necessary for subjects to respond successfully to test suggestions. This assumption is fallacious. A series of experiments (Barber & Calverley, 1962, 1963b, 1963c), which are summarized elsewhere (Barber, 1965a, 1969b), indicate that a substantial proportion of subjects are very responsive to test suggestions when a "hypnotic induction procedure" is not administered. Let us briefly summarize these experiments.

The 186 college students who participated in these experiments were randomly assigned to one of three experimental conditions. One-third of the subjects were exposed to a standardized 15-minute "hypnotic induction procedure" that focused on repeated suggestions of relaxation, drowsiness, and sleep. Another third of the subjects were exposed for one minute to "task motivational instructions" that contained the following information: (a) the subject's performance would depend on his willingness to try to imagine vividly and to experience those things that would be described to him; (b) previous subjects were able to imagine vividly and to have the experiences that were suggested when they put aside notions that this was a difficult or silly thing to do; and (c) if they tried to imagine to the best of their ability, they would experience interesting things and would not be wasting either their own or the experimenter's time. The remaining one-third of the subjects (controls) were simply told to try to imagine those things that would be suggested. Immediately after receiving either the hypnotic induction procedure, the task motivational instructions, or the control instruction, each subject was tested on response to the following eight test suggestions, which comprise the Barber Suggestibility Scale: the subject's right arm is becoming heavy and is moving down; his left arm is becoming light and is moving up; he cannot take his clasped hands apart; he is becoming extremely thirsty; he cannot say his name; his body is stuck to the chair and he cannot get up; when the experiment is over, he will cough automatically when he hears a click; and, when the experiment is over, he will forget that he was given the suggestion that his arm was becoming light and was moving up.[1]

The results were as follows: 53% of the subjects exposed to the hypnotic induction procedure, 60% of those exposed to the task motivational instructions, and 16% of the control subjects showed a rather high level of response to the test suggestions (responding overtly to at least 5 of the 8 items on the Barber Suggestibility Scale and stating that they subjectively experienced at least 5 of the suggested effects). These results indicate that (a) some subjects (about 1 of 6) show a rather high level of response to test suggestions when they are tested without any special preliminaries (under a control condition), (b) both task motivational instructions and a hypnotic induction procedure raise responsiveness to test suggestions above the base (control) level, and (c) task motivational instructions are about as effective as a hypnotic induction procedure in raising response to test suggestions (cf. Matheus, 1973; Powers, 1972).

However, in these studies, the hypnotic induction procedure was standardized—was administered in the same way for 15 minutes to all subjects—and focused on repeated suggestions of relaxation, drowsiness, and sleep. Skilled hypnotists rarely administer *standardized* induction procedures and they do not simply repeat to the subject over and over that he is becoming relaxed, drowsy, and sleepy. On the contrary, skilled hypnotists vary their induction procedures to fit each subject's ongoing experiences. Furthermore, skilled hypnotists include task motivational instructions in their induction procedures and, in addition, include many other factors, such as "coupling suggestions with actual events" and "preventing or reinterpreting the subject's failure to pass suggestions," which we shall discuss in this chapter.

Hypnotists claim there is an art to "hypnotizing," which depends primarily on varying the suggestions and instructions that are included in induction procedures so that they are congruent with the ongoing experiences of the subject. We shall discuss the art of "hypnotizing" in this chapter and also in the next one. In this chapter, we shall discuss how hypnotists can vary their induction procedures in order to maximize their subjects' responsiveness to test suggestions. In the next chapter, we shall explain how induction procedures give rise to a "hypnotic" appearance, changes in body feelings, and reports of having been hypnotized.

VARIABLES THAT AUGMENT RESPONSIVENESS TO TEST SUGGESTIONS

The first column in Table 1 lists eight variables that are associated with induction procedures (Barber & De Moor, 1972).[2] When administering induction procedures, hypnotists typically utilize some of these variables—for instance, they define the situation as hypnosis, ask the subject to keep his eyes closed, and repeatedly suggest that the subject is becoming relaxed, drowsy, and sleepy. Other variables—for example, removing fears and misconceptions and coupling suggestions with actual events—may or may not be included in induction procedures but they should be if the hypnotist intends to maximize the subject's responsiveness to test suggestions.

As shown in Table 1, column 2, we see the eight antecedent variables associated with induction procedures as giving rise to positive attitudes, motivations, and expectancies toward being "hypnotized" or responding to suggestions. As will be discussed in Chapter 5, a "positive attitude" is present when the subject views being "hypnotized" or responding to suggestions as worthwhile or valuable; a "positive motivation" is present when he right now, in the immediate test situation, wants to be or tries to be "hypnotized" or to have the experiences that are suggested; and a "positive expectancy" is present when he believes that he himself can be "hypnotized" or can have the experiences that are suggested. Also, as shown in Table 1, column 3, positive attitudes, motivations, and expectancies tend to give rise to a willingness to think and imagine with the themes that are suggested. And, as shown in Table 1, column 4, when the subject thinks and imagines with the suggestions, he tends to show high responsiveness to test suggestions. Let us first relate each of the eight variables listed in Table 1, column 1, to responsiveness to test suggestions.

Variable 1. Defining the Situation as Hypnosis

Induction procedures explicitly or implicitly define the situation to the subject as hypnosis. Two experiments (Barber & Calverley, 1964f, 1965a) have shown that this factor—simply labeling the situation as *hypnosis*—is sufficient by itself to enhance responsiveness to test suggestions. In both experiments, the subjects were randomly assigned to one of two experimental treatments. Sub-

Table 1. Induction Variables, Mediating Variables, and Consequent Variables

(1)	(2)	(3)	(4)
Variables Associated with Induction Procedures	Mediating Variables— First Set	Mediating Variables— Second Set	Consequent Variables
1. Defining the situation as hypnosis	Positive attitudes, motivations, and expectancies	Thinking and imagining with the suggestions	1. Responsiveness to test suggestions (for arm levitation, limb or body rigidity, age regression, analgesia, hallucination, amnesia, etc.)
2. Removing fears and misconceptions			2. "Hypnotic" appearance
3. Securing cooperation			3. Changes in body feelings
4. Asking the subject to keep his eyes closed			4. Reports of having been hypnotized
5. Suggesting relaxation, sleep, and hypnosis			
6. Elaborating and varying the wording and tone of suggestions			
7. Coupling suggestions with actual events			
8. Preventing or reinterpreting the subject's failure to pass suggestions			

jects assigned to one treatment were told individually that they were participating in a hypnosis experiment, and those assigned to the other treatment were told individually that they were control subjects. After the situation had been defined in these different ways, subjects assigned to both treatments were treated *identically*; that is, they were tested immediately on response to the eight standardized test suggestions of the Barber Suggestibility Scale. In each of the two studies, subjects who were told that they were in a hypnosis experiment showed a small but statistically significant gain in suggestibility as compared to those who were told that they were control subjects.

The results of the two experiments summarized above raise an important question: When other factors are held constant, why are subjects on the average somewhat more responsive to test suggestions when the situation is defined to them as "hypnosis" rather than as a "control" experiment? One important factor that seems to be involved is subjects' assumptions about hypnosis. For more than a century, practically everyone has assumed that subjects in a hypnosis experiment manifest a high level of responsiveness to test suggestions. Subjects participating in present-day experiments, who are typically college students, accept this assumption (Dorcus, Brintnall, & Case, 1941; London, 1961). Consequently, when present-day subjects are told that they are in a hypnosis experiment, they may construe this to mean that (a) they are in a special kind of situation in which a high level of responsiveness to test suggestions is desired and expected and (b) if they do not try to experience those things that the hypnotist suggests, they will be considered poor or uncooperative subjects and the hypnotist will be disappointed. On the other hand, when subjects are told that they are in the "control" group, they may not necessarily expect to manifest a high level of responsiveness to test suggestions of the type traditionally associated with the word "hypnosis."

Variable 2. Removing Fears and Misconceptions

Although simply defining the situation as hypnosis is sufficient to produce a significant enhancement of responsiveness to test suggestions in most subjects, the hypnotist typically attempts to enhance further the subject's readiness to respond. Before beginning his more formal procedures, the well-trained hypnotist administers a "preinduction education" that aims in part to remove fears and misconceptions.

Some subjects have inhibitory fears about hypnotism. Authors such as Hartland (1966), Weitzenhoffer (1957), and Wolberg (1948) discuss in detail what should be done in such cases. The hypnotist should first try to find the reasons for the fears and misconceptions and should then try to remove them. Since positive attitudes and motivations are necessary for the subject to participate actively in the production of the desired responses, these authors advocate that, before beginning the more formal procedures, the hypnotist should give a reassuring talk concerning the usual misgivings, false ideas, and prejudices about hypnotism. Hartland (1966) pointed out that most failures "are due to lack of adequate preparation of the subject and lack of adequate discussion before induction is attempted" (p. 20). This "preparation" or "preinduction education" should include attempts to obviate fears that revolve around loss of will power or becoming unaware or unconscious. The importance of this kind of "pre-induction education" has been demonstrated in recent studies by Cronin, Spanos, and Barber (1971), Diamond (1972), and Macvaugh (1969). Each of these studies showed that subjects are more responsive to test suggestions after the hypnotist has given favorable information about hypnosis with the intention of removing inhibitory fears and misconceptions.

Variable 3. Securing Cooperation

Even when the subject's fears and misconceptions have been minimized, additional measures are usually needed to secure a high level of motivation and cooperation. Wolberg (1948) noted that subjects' responsiveness in a hypnotic situation depends on their motivation to be hypnotized: "Before hypnosis is attempted, the physician must build up motivations for hypnosis" (p. 111). Hartland (1966) also emphasized that the subject "must either want to comply with the suggestions of the hypnotist or must feel that, regardless of his own will, he cannot resist" (p. 18).

How do hypnotists go about enhancing the subject's motivation and securing his cooperation? The hypnotist may explicitly ask the subject for his cooperation. He may inform the subject that his willingness to imagine vividly or to think with those things that are suggested is crucial. He may also inform the subject that he will have interesting experiences if he cooperates. As noted at the beginning of this chapter, a series of experiments indicated that these elements of the "preinduction education" are very important in heightening responsiveness to test suggestions. In these experiments, the subjects were given a set of task motivational instructions that asked them to cooperate, to try to experience those things that would be suggested, and to try to imagine to the best of their ability. In addition, the subjects were told that, if they cooperated and tried to imagine, they would find it easy to have interesting experiences. The task motivational instructions were effective in producing a significant enhancement of suggestibility. In fact, as we noted previously, the task motivational instructions were generally as effective in raising responsiveness to test suggestions as a standardized 15-minute "hypnotic induction" that focused on repeated suggestions of relaxation, drowsiness, sleep, and hypnosis.

Variable 4. Asking the Subject to Keep his Eyes Closed

At the beginning of the formal induction procedure, the hypnotist either asks the subject to close his eyes or suggests that the eyes are becoming heavy and are closing. Typically, the subject then keeps his eyes closed during the remainder of the session. Keeping the eyes closed may play a role in removing visual distractions, in enhancing the subject's ability to imagine vividly, and in augmenting responsiveness to some types of test suggestions—for example, suggestions for age regression. It also appears that keeping the eyes closed may be *necessary* to respond to certain kinds of suggestions, such as suggestions to have a dream on a specified topic.

However, whether or not the subject's eyes are closed may not significantly affect responsiveness to more "simple" or "motoric" test suggestions such as those that suggest arm heaviness, arm levitation, or body immobility (Barber & Calverley, 1965a). Further research is clearly needed to ascertain more precisely what types of test suggestions are more easily carried out and what types are not affected when the subject keeps his eyes closed.

Variable 5. Suggesting Relaxation, Sleep, and Hypnosis

Most present-day induction procedures include repeated suggestions of relaxation, drowsiness, sleep, and hypnosis (henceforth labeled *relaxation-sleep-hypnosis suggestions*). An important question for theories of hypnotism is whether such suggestions heighten responsiveness to test suggestions. If so, why?

Earlier in this chapter, while discussing variable 1, we stated that, when other variables are held constant, subjects are more responsive to test suggestions if they are told that they are participating in a hypnosis experiment rather than in a control experiment. In the present section, we shall discuss a supplementary finding: When the situation is defined to all subjects as hypnosis, the subjects are more responsive to test suggestions if they are also exposed to relaxation-sleep-hypnosis suggestions.

In four experiments (Barber & Calverley, 1965a, 1965b—Experiments 1 and 2; Starr & Tobin, 1970), subjects who were randomly assigned to one experimental condition were tested individually on the Barber Suggestibility Scale after they had been told that they were participating in a hypnosis experiment; in addition, they had been exposed to repeated relaxation-sleep-hypnosis suggestions (e.g., "Relax completely . . . breathing regularly and deeply . . . drowsy and sleepy. . . . Soon you will be deeply asleep, but you will have no trouble hearing me . . . deep, sound sleep . . . deepest trance . . .). Subjects who were randomly assigned to another experimental condition were tested individually on the Barber Suggestibility Scale immediately after they were told simply that they were participating in a hypnosis experiment—without being exposed to relaxation-sleep-hypnosis suggestions. Each of the studies showed that, when other factors are held constant, repeated relaxation-sleep-hypnosis suggestions produce a statistically significant gain in suggestibility, which is above that found when subjects are told only that they are participating in a hypnosis experiment.

Why do subjects generally show a higher level of responsiveness to test suggestions when they are given repeated suggestions of relaxation, drowsiness, sleep, and hypnosis? At least part of the gain in suggestibility associated with relaxation-sleep-hypnosis suggestions appears to be due to the special effectiveness of these kinds of suggestions in defining the situation to the subject as "truly hypnosis," which tends to produce more positive attitudes, motivations, and expectancies toward the situation and a willingness to think and imagine with the suggestions. This interpretation is based on the following interrelated considerations:

The situation is not very effectively defined as hypnosis to present-day subjects when they are told simply that they are participating in a hypnosis experiment and the hypnotist does *not* go on to say the kinds of things that hypnotists are expected to say—for example, if he does not repeatedly suggest that the subject is becoming relaxed, drowsy, and sleepy. We have observed that under these conditions some subjects seem to doubt that the situation is "truly hypnosis," and they typically state afterwards that the experimenter was not a good hypnotist. However, we have also observed that subjects' doubts as to whether they are actually participating in a hypnosis experiment are effectively removed when the experimenter goes on to suggest repeatedly that they are becoming relaxed and drowsy and are entering a state of sleep or hypnosis. Now, when the situation is *effectively* defined as hypnosis, most subjects appear to be aware that, if they resist and if they do not try to think and imagine with the themes of the suggestions, they will negate the purpose of the experiment, the experimenter's time and effort will be wasted, the experimenter will be disappointed, and they will be considered poor or uncooperative subjects. Stated somewhat differently, when the situation is effectively defined as hypnosis—that is, when the subjects perceive the situation as unusual, different, and special (as "truly hypnosis")—they concomitantly tend to perceive it as one in which high responsiveness to suggestions is desired and expected and in which they should cooperate by trying to think and imagine with the themes that are suggested.

The traditional interpretation. The above interpretation is markedly different from the traditional one concerning how relaxation-sleep-hypnosis suggestions produce heightened suggestibility. The traditional interpretation postulates that repeated suggestions of relaxation, drowsiness, sleep, and hypnosis raise responsiveness to test suggestions because they produce relaxation and a special state ("hypnotic trance"). However, the following three sets of data seem to contradict the traditional interpretation:

1. Repeated suggestions of relaxation, drowsiness, sleep, and hypnosis are effective in producing physical relaxation (as measured by physiological indices such as increased regularity of respiration and reduced forehead muscle tension) in *some* subjects (Barber, 1961c; Barber & Hahn, 1963). However, this induced relaxation usually disappears when suggestions are given that require the subject to be active—e.g., suggestions for heightened strength and endurance or suggestions to try to bend an "immovable" arm (Barber & Coules, 1959). Even though the induced relaxation *is no longer present* when test suggestions are given that involve effort or activity, the subjects nevertheless tend to show a heightened level of responsiveness to the test suggestions.

2. If subjects who have been given repeated relaxation-sleep-hypnosis suggestions show a high level of responsiveness to test suggestions while they appear to be relaxed or in a "hypnotic trance," they can be told: "Be alert and awake. Stop being relaxed and sleepy. Stop appearing to be in a trance, but respond to my suggestions." Or they can be told: "In a moment the experiment will be over and you will wake up. When you are awake, you will respond to all of the suggestions that I will give you. Now, 1, 2, 3, wake up. The experiment is over." If the experimenter then goes ahead and gives test suggestions, many of the subjects will continue to respond to the suggestions even though they now do not show signs of relaxation or "hypnotic trance" (Barber, 1962b).

3. As noted at the beginning of this chapter, if it is made clear to subjects that they are in a special situation in which they are expected to respond to suggestions, it is not necessary to administer relaxation-sleep-hypnosis suggestions in order to elicit a high level of responsiveness to test suggestions. In fact, some of the early mesmerists and hypnotists did not administer suggestions of relaxation, drowsiness, and sleep. They made "passes" over the subject's body and gave suggestions in a situation of high expectancy, but they did not suggest to the subject that he was becoming relaxed and was entering a state of sleep (Binet & Fèrè, 1888; Darnton, 1968).

In brief, it appears more likely that repeated relaxation-sleep-hypnosis suggestions tend to raise responsiveness to test suggestions not because they produce relaxation or a special state ("hypnotic trance") but because they define the situation to the subject as "truly hypnosis"—as a situation in which high responsiveness to suggestions is desired and expected and in which they should try to think and imagine with the themes that are suggested.

Variable 6. Elaborating and Varying the Wording and Tone of Suggestions

The precise wording of the test suggestions also appears to play an important role in determining the subject's response. Wolberg (1972) has correctly pointed out that suggestions are usually given in terms of "word pictures." For instance, he writes:

> . . . if a hypnotist wishes to suggest that a subject prone to chilliness will feel warm, he might propose that the subject picture himself in a room with the windows closed and the heat turned on. The subject is not told that he will lose his tension and become relaxed. Instead, he may be asked to visualize himself lying on the beach in a comfortable position, inhaling deeply and feeling free from care [p. 91].

Hypnotists have learned through practice that a simple suggestion that something is occurring—e.g., "You cannot bend your arm," "Your hand is insensitive," "You are six years of age"—is rarely effective. To produce arm rigidity, hand anesthesia, or age regression, more elaborate suggestions are needed. For instance, to produce arm rigidity, the trained hypnotist will intone a series of suggestions such as:

> As I stroke your arm . . . you will feel that it is becoming much stiffer and straighter. The stiffness is increasing. . . . You can feel all the muscles tightening up . . . stiffer and straighter . . . it is beginning to feel just as stiff and rigid as a steel poker. . . . Picture a steel poker in your mind . . . you will feel that your arm has become just as stiff and rigid as that steel poker . . . [Hartland, 1966, pp. 81-82].

Similarly, the trained hypnotist will not simply suggest that a hand is insensitive; instead, he will give more extended and elaborate suggestions such as "Novocain has been injected into the hand. . . . You feel the numbness spreading. . . . The hand is dull, numb, and insensitive. . . . It is a piece of rubber, a lump of matter, without feeling, without sensation. . . ." Along similar lines, the trained hypnotist will not simply suggest to the subject that he is six years old; instead, he will give more elaborate suggestions intended to induce the subject to focus his thoughts on the past, to imagine vividly events that occurred at the age of six, and to put aside thoughts about the present. In fact, learning to be an effective hypnotist consists primarily of learning the art of giving suggestions that include elaborate "word pictures" or descriptive imagery.

Some of the elaboration of suggestions involves guiding the subject to carry out *goal-directed imagining*—that is, to imagine a situation which, if it actually occurred, would tend to produce the suggested behavior. Test suggestions are often worded in such a way as to produce goal-directed imagining (Spanos, 1971). For instance, a test suggestion for arm heaviness is typically worded as follows: ". . . Imagine you are holding something heavy in your hand. . . . Now the hand and arm feel heavy as if the [imagined] weight were pressing down . . . and as it feels heavier and heavier the hand and arm begin to move down . . ." (Weitzenhoffer & Hilgard, 1962). This test suggestion aims to elicit goal-directed imagining in that, if the situation described by the suggestion were to occur objectively (if the subject held a heavy weight in his hand), the arm would feel heavy and would tend to move downward. In Chapter 6, we shall describe recent experiments (Spanos, 1971; Spanos & Barber, 1972, Spanos & Ham, 1973) which indicate that the stimulation of goal-directed imagining is an important variable in enhancing responsiveness to test suggestions and in producing the feeling that the overt responses occurred involuntarily.

Whether the suggestions are worded permissively or authoritatively may also be important. Two recent studies indicate that permissively worded suggestions tend to be more effective than those that are worded authoritatively. More subjects showed apparent amnesia—that is, testified that they had forgotten specified material—when they were given permissive suggestions ("Try to forget") rather than authoritative suggestions ("You will forget") (Barber & Calverley, 1966b). Similarly, when awakened at night during rapid eye movement (REM) periods, there was a tendency for more subjects to testify that they were dreaming about a suggested topic if they had received a permissive suggestion ("Try to think and to dream about [the selected topic] all through the night. . . .") rather than if they had received an authoritatively worded suggestion ("You will think about and dream about [the selected topic] all through the night") (Barber, 1969b, pp. 66-67).

Of course, the suggestions should be phrased in such a way that they are clear to the subject. The subject cannot respond to words he does not understand. Gindes (1951, p. 104) illustrated this point in an amusing way. A hypnotist repeatedly suggested that the subject was becoming more and more lethargic. After an hour of futile effort, the subject opened his eyes and asked, "What is 'lethargic' anyway?"

In addition to the wording of the test suggestions, hypnotists also stress the importance of vocal characteristics such as intonations, inflections, and volume. Hartland (1966) has placed heavy emphasis on these aspects of the suggestions and has given many examples of the following variations in the proper use of vocal expressions: (a) alterations in the volume of the voice, (b) changes in the inflection and modulation of the voice, (c) changes in the rate of delivery, (d) stressing of particular words, and (e) insertion of suitable pauses between suggested ideas.

Although we agree with Hartland that the vocal qualities of suggestions play a role in determining the subject's response, this variable has not as yet been subjected to intensive experimental evaluation. In fact, we know of only one experiment that assessed the effect on suggestibility of variations in the hypnotist's tone of voice. In this experiment (Barber & Calverley, 1964b), the eight test-suggestions from the Barber Suggestibility Scale were administered to all of the subjects. However, half of the subjects received the suggestions in a lackadaisical tone of voice and the others received the same suggestions in a firm, forceful tone. A higher level of response to the test suggestions was elicited when the suggestions were presented forcefully rather than lackadaisically. These results were presumably due to the following: a forceful tone reflects an attitude of confidence on the part of the experimenter, which conveys to the subject that what the experimenter suggests ought to happen. On the other hand, a lackadaisical tone reflects a nonconfident or an uninvolved attitude on the part of the experimenter, and this uninvolved attitude presumably transfers to the subject.

In brief, it appears that variations in the wording and tone of test suggestions play a role in determining the subject's responsiveness. However, further research is needed to specify more precisely the specific variations in the phrasing and vocal characteristics of suggestions that exert effects on specific kinds of responses.

Variable 7. Coupling Suggestions with Actual Events

Trained hypnotists try to couple their suggestions with events that are actually occurring in the situation. The underlying principle involved here has been formulated by Hartland (1966) as follows: "You should always couple an effect that you want to produce with one that the subject is actually experiencing at the moment" (p. 35). Spiegel (1959) refers to this variable as ". . . the art of induction . . . tacitly implying that the phenomena are due to the signal of the hypnotist."

As Weitzenhoffer (1957, p. 273) has noted, Erickson's "specialized techniques" (cf. Erickson, 1967) seem to pivot around this variable in three interrelated ways: (a) whatever technique is employed is adapted to the ongoing behavioral activities of the subject; (b) whatever behavior the subject manifests is interpreted as a successful response (leading the subject to believe he is responding appropriately whether this is actually true or not); and (c) suggestions are given that anticipate behaviors or experiences that will occur naturally. The major purpose of these techniques appears to be to lead the subject to believe that he is responding well to suggestions and thus may expect that he will continue to respond well.

Gindes (1951) referred to this variable as an "innocent artifice" and commented as follows: "The therapist's words must closely follow the subject's actions without his growing aware of it. The interaction of these two factors leads the subject to believe that he is following the operator's suggestions, although the reverse is true" (p. 90).

Let us now briefly glance at some of the techniques that attempt to use actually occurring, nonsuggested events to enhance suggestibility.

When using the Eye-Fixation technique, the hypnotist asks the subject to look at an object that is held a little above the eyes. While the subject stares at the fixation object, a strain upon his eyes tends to occur. Suggestions that the eyes are becoming tired and are closing are timed to coincide with the natural fatigue that occurs. In one variant of the Postural-Sway technique, the subject is asked to stand with his eyes closed and, since no one stands perfectly still when the eyes are closed, the trained hypnotist detects the rhythm of the swayings. The suggestions of sway are then timed to coincide with the naturally occurring sway (Watkins, 1949). When using the Metronome technique, the hypnotist suggests heaviness of the eyes while the subject focuses his gaze at a blinking light and listens to the monotonous sound of the metronome. The latter factors—gazing at the light and listening to the metronome—tend to produce a feeling of eye-heaviness. Similarly, in Drug Hypnosis, the drugs that are used tend to produce drowsiness, narcosis, or confusion, and the hypnotist times his suggestions of drowsiness to coincide with the chemically induced effects (Weitzenhoffer, 1957, pp. 255-263).

Variable 8. Preventing or Reinterpreting the Subject's Failure to Pass Suggestions

Hypnotists at times challenge the subject to overcome a suggested effect. For instance, the subject may be challenged to open his eyes while suggestions are given that he cannot do so. If the subject overcomes the challenge and opens his eyes, his expectancy that he can successfully pass test suggestions will probably be reduced and he will tend to be less responsive to subsequent test suggestions. Consequently, skillful hypnotists at times phrase the challenge in such a way that the subject will not have the opportunity to discover that he has failed a test suggestion. For example, instead of directly suggesting to the subject that he cannot open his eyes, the hypnotist might give suggestions as follows: "Your eyes are stuck tight . . . so tight that *if* you tried to open them *you could not*. But you will *not* try to open them. *You have no desire* to open your eyes, but only want to sleep deeper" (Weitzenhoffer, 1957, p. 214). Along similar lines, Wolberg (1972, p. 108) has noted that even if the subject fails a test suggestion, he should be told: "You are responding well to suggestions." London (1967) has stated the underlying principle in this way: "The thrust of the patter most commonly used in inductions therefore deliberately soft-pedals the occurrence of failure on the subject's part by variously justifying it, approving it, denying it, or retrospectively confusing the issue so that the subject cannot be sure he has failed at all" (p. 70).

Although preventing or reinterpreting the subject's failure to pass suggestions appears to be important, this factor has not as yet been tested experimentally. Further research is needed to determine the precise effects on suggestibility of preventing the subject from failing test suggestions and of reinterpreting failures as nonfailures.

Supplementary Variables

We have listed eight variables associated with induction procedures that tend to raise responsiveness to test suggestions. This list is not exhaustive. Many other variables might also play a role in some types of induction procedures. For instance, suggestibility might be enhanced in some cases if the hypnotist reinforces the subject from time to time for desired responses by stating: "Good," "Fine," or "Excellent" (Bullard, 1973). Additional variables that are not an integral part of induction procedures might also affect the subject's responsiveness, such as the hypnotist's confident attitude and his prestige and personality characteristics (Greenberg & Land, 1971; Powers, 1972; Small & Kramer, 1969). Responsiveness to test suggestions might also be at a higher level in those subjects who are acquainted with or have formed a close relationship with the hypnotist prior to the hypnotic session (Kramer, 1969; Richman, 1965; Wilson, 1967). Also, the subject's responsiveness to test suggestions is affected by the amount and kind of prior practice or training that he has received in responding to suggestions (Barber, Ascher, & Mavroides, 1971; Barber & Calverley, 1966c; Cooper, Banford, Schubot, & Tart, 1967). If the subject receives practice in responding to *identical* test suggestions in a series of sessions, he tends to get bored, to find the situation less and less interesting, and to show a continual reduction in responsiveness (Barber & Calverley, 1966c). On the other hand, if the subject is given practice in a series of sessions in responding to a variety of *different* types of suggestions, he tends to find the sessions interesting and tends to improve his response (Barber, Ascher, & Mavroides, 1971). Further research is needed to determine (a) to what degree each of the eight variables, and also other supplementary variables, facilitate suggestibility, (b) which variables, when applied in combination, have an additive effect, and (c) what combination of variables are sufficient to maximize responsiveness.

SUMMARY

Which of the many variables associated with induction procedures are effective in enhancing responsiveness to test suggestions? Eight variables were delineated in this chapter that appear to have this suggestibility-enhancing effect: (a) defining the situation as hypnosis, (b) removing fears and misconceptions, (c) securing cooperation, (d) asking the subject to keep his eyes closed, (e) suggesting relaxation, sleep, and hypnosis, (f) elaborating and varying the wording and tone of suggestions, (g) coupling suggestions with actual events, and (h) preventing or reinterpreting the subject's failure to pass suggestions. An underlying contention in the chapter was that the eight variables augment suggestibility because they give rise to positive attitudes, motivations, and expectancies toward responding to suggestions or being "hypnotized," which in turn give rise to a willingness to think and imagine with the themes that are suggested.

NOTES

[1] Since the Barber Suggestibility Scale will be often cited in this text, a more detailed account of the scale together with methods for scoring the subjects' responses is presented in Appendix A, which is found at the end of the volume.

[2] We are deeply indebted to Dr. Wilfried De Moor, University of Tilburg, The Netherlands, for invaluable assistance in conceptualizing the variables that are associated with induction procedures.

* * *

Wolberg extract is from Wolberg, L.R. *Hypnosis: Is it for You?* New York: Harcourt Brace Jovanovich, Inc., 1972.

Hartland extract is from Hartland, J. *Medical and Dental Hypnosis and its Clinical Applications.* Reproduced from the second edition, 1971, Balliere Tindall, London.

CHAPTER 4

Producing Other "Hypnotic" Effects ("Hypnotic" Appearance, Changes in Body Feelings, and Reports of Having Been Hypnotized)

In addition to raising responsiveness to test suggestions, induction procedures also tend to give rise to three additional phenomena—a "hypnotic" appearance, changes in body feelings, and reports of having been hypnotized. From the traditional viewpoint, the latter three phenomena have been considered to be indices of a "hypnotic trance," and the "trance" has been regarded as a critical factor in producing heightened responsiveness to test suggestions. However, these phenomena can be parsimoniously explained without making use of the "trance state" notion. Empirical findings suggest that the "hypnotic" appearance, the changes in body feelings, and the reports of having been hypnotized are due, primarily, to suggestions and instructions included in induction procedures and they are *not* necessary, although they may be helpful, in producing heightened responsiveness to test suggestions. Let us again look at induction procedures to ascertain which antecedent variables give rise to a "hypnotic" appearance, changes in body feelings, and reports of having been hypnotized.

"HYPNOTIC" APPEARANCE

As Weitzenhoffer (1957, pp. 210-211) and other writers have pointed out, subjects who have been exposed to an induction procedure typically manifest a "hypnotic" appearance. For instance, they appear limp or relaxed, they lack spontaneity, and they move their limbs or body very slowly (psychomotor retardation). Also, when asked to open their eyes, they at times show a fixed stare (a "trance stare"). Which of the many variables included in induction procedures give rise to a "hypnotic" appearance?

An experiment by Barber and Calverley (1969) indicated that the "hypnotic" appearance—as indicated by limpness-relaxation, lack of spontaneity, psychomotor retardation, and a "fixed stare"—is due in part to asking the subject to keep his eyes closed during the experiment (variable 4 in Table 1, p. 20). The same experiment also indicated that an even greater proportion of subjects manifest a "hypnotic" appearance if they not only keep their eyes closed but, in addition, are given repeated suggestions of relaxation, drowsiness, and sleep or are told to put themselves in hypnosis.

Since the "hypnotic" appearance is primarily due to suggestions for relaxation, drowsiness, sleep, and/or hypnosis that are given to the subject while his eyes are closed, one wonders whether a "hypnotic" appearance or the variables leading to it are essential for the subject to manifest a high level of responsiveness to test suggestions for limb rigidity, body immobility, analgesia, age regression, amnesia, and the like. This does not seem to be the case.

The "hypnotic" appearance can be removed by suggestions or instructions and the subject can continue to show a high level of responsiveness to test suggestions. For instance, several years ago, one of the authors (T.X.B.) carried out the following unpublished study with eight responsive subjects. The subjects were first exposed to a "hypnotic induction procedure" that focused on repeated relaxation-sleep-hypnosis suggestions. The subjects manifested a "hypnotic" appearance and also responded to test suggestions for arm heaviness, arm levitation, inability ot take their clasped hands apart, and hallucination of thirst. Next, the subjects were told to be awake and alert, to stop appearing as if they were in a trance, but to continue to remain responsive to test suggestions. The subjects remained highly responsive to test suggestions for inability to say their name, body immobility, and selective amnesia, but they no longer showed a "hypnotic" appearance; in fact, they appeared as alert and awake as any other normal individual.

Instructing subjects to be alert is not the sole means of removing the "hypnotic" appearance. As stated in Chapter 3, it may also be removed (a) by administering test suggestions that require activity, effort, or alertness—for instance, test suggestions for heightened strength and endurance—or (b) by instructing the subject to respond to the test suggestions that he will receive in the postexperimental period and then stating: "Wake up—the experiment is over" (Barber, 1958, 1962b). After the "hypnotic" appearance has been removed by these suggestions or instructions, the subject may continue to manifest a high level of responsiveness to test suggestions. In other words, the hypnotist can first give suggestions—for example, relaxation-sleep-hypnosis suggestions—that tend to produce a "hypnotic" appearance, and then he can give suggestions to remove the "hypnotic" appearance; neither the suggestions that give rise to the "hypnotic" appearance nor those that remove it necessarily affect the subject's responsiveness to test suggestions.

Of course, a high level of responsiveness to test suggestions can be elicited without first inducing a "hypnotic" appearance. If subjects are not asked to close their eyes and are not given relaxation-drowsiness-sleep suggestions, many subjects will show a high level of responsiveness to test suggestions, especially if the experimenter implements some of the other variables that are commonly included in induction procedures—e.g., securing cooperation, coupling suggestions with actual events, and preventing or reinterpreting the subject's failure to pass suggestions (Arons, 1961; Barber, 1969b, 1970, 1972; Barber & Calverley, 1963a; Dalal, 1966; Klopp, 1961; Meeker & Barber, 1971; Nichols, 1968; Wells, 1924).

CHANGES IN BODY FEELINGS

Subjects who have been exposed to an induction procedure typically report several kinds of changes in body feelings. For instance, a subject may report that he felt that his arm was rising involuntarily or that his hand felt numb and insensitive. Since these kinds of changes in body feelings are found when the subject has received test suggestions for arm levitation or of hand anesthesia, they can be viewed as direct responses to test suggestions.

However, subjects also report changes in body feelings that have not been directly suggested by the hypnotist. For instance, Gill and Brenman (1959, pp. 13-19) noted that a substantial proportion of subjects who have been exposed to an induction procedure report changes in the size of the body or body parts, "disappearance" of the body or parts of the body, changes in equilibrium such as giddiness or dizziness, changes in feelings of reality ("things seemed unreal"), changes in experienced temperature (feeling either very hot or very cold), and changes in the way the hypnotist's voice is experienced (as either very near or very far). An experiment by Barber and Calverley (1969) indicated that these kinds of changes in body feelings are due in part to variable 4 (keeping the eyes closed for a period of time) and in part to variable 5 (receiving suggestions of relaxation, drowsiness, sleep and/or hypnosis). In this experiment, subjects who had *not* had prior experience with "hypnosis" were assigned to one of three experimental groups. Subjects assigned to one group (Induction group) were individually exposed to repeated suggestions of relaxation, drowsiness, sleep, and hypnosis and to a series of test suggestions. Subjects assigned to a second group (Place-Yourself-in-Hypnosis group) were asked individually to put themselves in hypnosis and, after five minutes had elapsed, were assessed on response to the same test suggestions. Subjects in a third group (a control group or a Close-Your-Eyes group) were individually asked to close their eyes and to await further instructions.[1] At the end of each individual session, each subject completed a rating scale that described changes in body feelings that might have occurred during the experiment. The results are presented in Table 2.

Table 2. Percentage of Subjects in Close-Your-Eyes, Induction, and Place-Yourself-in-Hypnosis Groups Reporting Changes in Body Feelings

	Close-Your-Eyes control group ($N = 55$)	Induction group ($N = 55$)	Place-Yourself-in-Hypnosis group ($N = 50$)
Changes in size of body or body parts	36	51	47
Changes in equilibrium (giddiness, dizziness, etc.)	66	85	76
Changes in experienced temperature (feeling either very hot or very cold)	34	36	42
"Disappearance" of body or body parts	4*	20	16
Changes in feelings of reality	26*	69	69
Changes in the way the experimenter's voice is experienced (as very near or very far)	34*	71	64

Note: The asterisk indicates that the percentage is significantly smaller than the other two percentages in the same *row* at the .05 level of confidence.

As Table 2 shows, subjects in the Close-Your-Eyes control group did not differ significantly from those in the Induction group or the Place-Yourself-in-Hypnosis group on three of the six items that assessed changes in body feelings (changes in the size of the body or body parts, changes in equilibrium, and changes in experienced temperature). The Close-Your-Eyes control group obtained lower scores than the other two groups on the remaining three items that assessed changes in body feelings ("disappearance" of the body or body parts, changes in feelings of reality, and changes in the way the experimenter's voice is experienced). It should be noted, however, that 26% of the subjects in the Close-Your-Eyes control group reported changes in feelings of reality and 34% testified that the experimenter's voice seemed either very near or very far away. Informal interviews suggested that the changes in body feelings reported by subjects in the Close-Your-Eyes control group may have been due to sitting quietly with eyes closed for a period of time while expecting *something* to occur but *not* due to their defining the situation as hypnosis or expecting hypnosis.

In brief, the study summarized above indicated that some of the changes in body feelings of the type described by Gill and Brenman (1959) may be due to the subject keeping his eyes closed for a period of time while expecting something to happen. However, the study also indicated that relaxation-sleep-hypnosis suggestions, or suggestions to enter hypnosis, also play an important role in producing these changes in body feelings. In fact, there is evidence indicating that relaxation *per se* can give rise to some changes in body feelings. For instance, Elmer Green and his collaborators (Green, Green, & Walters, 1970; Green, Walters, Green, & Murphy, 1969) used the following procedure to train subjects to achieve profound relaxation: the subjects repeated to themselves phrases such as, "My ankles, my knees, my hips feel heavy and relaxed," while they simultaneously received biofeedback information that helped to produce relaxation by reducing muscle tension, increasing the percentage of low-voltage alpha rhythm from the brain, and increasing the temperature of a hand (cf. Barber, DiCara, Kamiya, Miller, Shapiro, & Stoyva, 1971a, 1971b). The subjects who achieved relaxation reported changes in body feelings such as, "I felt I was floating above the chair," ". . . it seems like there was some kind of force on the inside, floating through my forehead out," "I'm not even sitting here. I feel like I'm just detached in some way," and "My arm feels like a bag of cement" or "like a ton of lead" or "like it is moving away from me" (Green, Green, & Walters, 1970, pp. 6-8).

Taken together, the data summarized above suggest that the changes in body feelings that are associated with induction procedures—e.g., changes in the size of the body or body parts, changes in equilibrium, and changes in feelings of reality—are due to several interrelated variables: keeping the eyes closed for a period of time; expecting something to happen or expecting changes in body feelings; receiving or giving oneself suggestions of relaxation, drowsiness, sleep, and hypnosis; achieving relaxation; and expectantly focusing on and magnifying the body feelings and sensations that are produced as one relaxes with his eyes closed while being told repeatedly that he is becoming relaxed, drowsy, and sleepy.

Do these changes in body feelings affect the subject's responsiveness to test suggestions? Although the changes in body feelings do not appear to have a *direct* effect, they may *indirectly* affect the subject's responsiveness to test suggestions by further heightening his expectancies. When the subject finds that he is experiencing changes in body feelings as he receives suggestions, his expectancy that he can be affected by suggestions may increase, and his heightened expectancy may enhance his responsiveness to subsequent test suggestions.

REPORTS OF HAVING BEEN HYPNOTIZED

Whether or not and to what degree subjects report that they were hypnotized is dependent on (a) whether the hypnotist states that they were hypnotized, (b) the wording of the questions that are submitted to them to elicit their reports, and (c) the degree of congruence between what they experienced and what they believe or expect that hypnosis involves. We shall discuss each of these variables in turn.

Effects of Cues from the Hypnotist on the Subjects' Report

An experiment presented by Barber, Dalal, and Calverley (1968) showed that whether subjects believe they were hypnotized is affected by cues from the hypnotist. In this experiment, 63 subjects were individually exposed to an induction procedure and to the Barber Suggestibility Scale. Next, the hypnotist spoke to each subject individually as follows: one-third of the subjects, selected at random, were told, "I observed you closely during the experiment and, from what I observed, you were hypnotized"; another third of the subjects, also selected at random, were told, "I observed you closely during the experiment and, from what I observed, you were not hypnotized." The hypnotist did not say anything to the remaining subjects. Since the subjects were exposed to the hypnotist's statements at random, the hypnotist's statements were not related to the subject's actual performance. Despite the fact that the three sets of subjects had performed very similarly during the experiment—for instance, they obtained practically identical scores on the Barber Suggestibility Scale—their postexperimental self-ratings of their hypnotic depth differed and were generally in line with the hypnotist's statements about their performance; that is, the subjects tended to say that they were (or were not) hypnotized if the hypnotist said that they were (or were not) hypnotized.

Although the cues from the hypnotist were explicit in the above experiment, there is reason to believe that the hypnotist may also transmit cues to his subjects through more subtle means, such as the manner in which he talks to them, the tone and inflections of his voice, and the type of questions that he asks (Barber, 1969b, 1973b; Barber & Calverley, 1964b; Barber & Silver, 1968a, 1968b; Rosenthal, 1968). In other words, subjects' reports pertaining to having been hypnotized were influenced by explicit cues from the hypnotist and, at times, may also be influenced by more subtle cues from the hypnotist.[2]

Wording of the Questions

The subjects' reports are also influenced by the wording of the questions they are asked. The importance of the wording of the questions was illustrated in another experiment by Barber, Dalal, and Calverley (1968). In this experiment, 53 subjects were exposed to an induction procedure and to the test suggestions that comprise the Stanford Hypnotic Susceptibility Scale.[3] Upon completion of the session, the subjects were randomly assigned to three groups and were individually asked the following questions:

Group A: "Did you experience the hypnotic state as basically similar to the waking state?"

Group B: "Did you experience the hypnotic state as basically different from the waking state?"

Group C: "Did you or did you not experience the hypnotic state as basically different from the waking state?"

Even though the subjects in Groups A, B, and C had performed in the same way during the session—for instance, their scores on the Stanford Hypnotic Susceptibility Scale were practically identical—the differently worded questions elicited markedly different replies. Only 17% of the subjects in Group A (who received the question that included the word *similar*) reported that the hypnotic state was experienced as basically *different* from the waking state. In contrast, 72% and 64% of the subjects in Groups B and C, respectively (who received the questions that included the word *different*), reported that the hypnotic state was experienced as basically *different* from the waking state. In brief, the subjects' reports pertaining to their experience of the hypnotic state were markedly influenced by the wording of the questions that were submitted to them.

We believe that the above findings were due to the following: Many subjects were willing to categorize their experiences in contradictory ways because their experiences were ambiguous or multifaceted and they did not know how to classify them. For instance, a subject could answer Yes to the question, "Did you experience the hypnotic state as basically different from the waking state?" because he experienced various suggested effects during the session. However, the same subject could also answer Yes to the antithetical question, "Did you experience the hypnotic state as basically similar to the waking state?" because he was aware of himself, of his role in the situation, and of extraneous events.

Congruence Between Experiences and Beliefs or Expectations Concerning "Hypnosis"

Barber and Calverley (1969) presented data indicating that subjects' reports pertaining to whether or not they were hypnotized are dependent on whether their experiences were harmonious with their beliefs and expectations of what hypnosis involves. Some highly responsive subjects who participated in this investigation gave reasons such as the following for believing that they were *not* truly hypnotized: they were aware of what they were doing, were aware of their surroundings, could think of extraneous things, could hear extraneous sounds, or did not have complete amnesia for the session. Although these subjects were highly responsive to test suggestions (and also showed a "hypnotic" appearance and reported changes in body feelings), they did not think they were truly hypnotized because their experiences were not harmonious with their beliefs and expectations of what true hypnosis is supposed to involve. They apparently believed that a person is truly hypnotized only if he is unaware of himself and his surroundings.

Although some subjects believe that hypnotized persons lose awareness, a study by Barber, Dalal, and Calverley (1968) indicated that (a) subjects typically believe that hypnosis involves relaxation and/or changes in body feelings and/or responsiveness to test suggestions and (b) they judge the degree to which they were hypnotized by noting the degree to which they experienced relaxation, changes in body feelings, or responsiveness to test suggestions. In this study, subjects who stated that they were hypnotized to a light, medium, or deep level were asked, "What basis did you use to judge your level of hypnotic depth?" Most of the replies could be classified into the three categories:

1. Some of the subjects stated that they judged their level of hypnotic depth from the degree to which they felt relaxed or sleepy. Of course, feeling relaxed or sleepy was a direct response to the suggestions for relaxation, drowsiness, and sleep that were used in the induction procedure.
2. Other subjects stated that they judged their degree of hypnosis on the basis of changes in body feelings. These changes in body feelings were of two types. One type was a direct response to test suggestions (for example, the feeling that a hand was rising involuntarily was a direct response to a test suggestion for hand levitation). A second type was similar to the kinds of changes in body feelings that have been specified by Gill and Brenman (for example, feelings of dizziness or giddiness, "disappearance" of the body or body parts, changes in experienced temperature, changes in feelings of reality, etc.). As stated previously in this chapter, these kinds of changes in body feelings appear to be due to several interacting variables, including (a) keeping the eyes closed for a period of time, (b) expecting something to happen or expecting changes in body feelings, (c) receiving or giving oneself suggestions of relaxation, drowsiness, sleep, and hypnosis, and (d) expectantly focusing on and magnifying the body feelings and sensations that are produced

when the eyes are closed and when suggestions of relaxation, drowsiness, sleep, and/or hypnosis are administered.

3. Most commonly, the subjects judged the degree to which they were hypnotized by observing the degree to which they experienced the effects that were suggested. Also, failure to experience some or all of the test suggestions was commonly given as a reason by the subjects for believing they were not hypnotized.

In line with the preceding paragraph, Gill and Brenman (1959) have noted that, when subjects state that they are hypnotized, they typically seem to mean that they are ready and willing to respond to suggestions. These authors documented this point, as follows:

> First, we would induce hypnosis in someone previously established as a "good" subject; then we would ask him how he knew he was in hypnosis . . . He might reply that he felt relaxed. Now we would suggest that the relaxation would disappear *but he would remain in hypnosis.* Then we would ask again how he knew he was in hypnosis. He might say because his arm "feels numb"—so again, we would suggest the disappearance of this sensation. We continued in this way until finally we obtained the reply, "I know I am in hypnosis because I *know* I will do what you tell me." This was repeated with several subjects, with the same results [p. 36].

Of course, the basic question here is: *Why* will the subject do what the experimenter tells him? Presumably, from the "hypnotic trance" viewpoint, the subject will do what he is told because he is in "hypnosis" or "trance" and, turning around circularly, the subject is judged to be in "hypnosis" or "trance" because he will do what he is told (Barber, 1964). From our own cognitive-behavioral perspective, the subject will do what he is told because he has positive attitudes, motivations, and expectancies toward the test situation that lead to a willingness to think and imagine with those things that are suggested.

An analogy. During recent years, investigators who adhere to the "hypnotic trance" formulation have more and more often been using the subject's report that he was hypnotized as a criterion for inferring the presence of "hypnotic trance." For instance, Conn and Conn (1967) stated that ". . . the subject and only the subject can report whether he is 'in' or 'out' of hypnosis" (p. 108). Similarly, Tart and Hilgard (1966) argued that the subject's "report that he feels hypnotized to some degree is primary data about the presence or absence of hypnosis, if not a criterion of hypnosis" (p. 253). However, from our viewpoint, serious methodological problems are involved in using the subject's report that he was hypnotized as a criterion for inferring the presence of a special state—"hypnotic trance." Let us clarify our viewpoint by presenting an analogy that compares the hypnotic subject's report that he was "hypnotized" with the report given by some individuals in preliterate cultures that they were "possessed."

For a number of years, anthropologists have been studying cultures that believe in spirit possession (Lewis, 1971). In many of these cultures, certain individuals, sometimes called *shamans*, behave in rather unusual ways. For example, they may maintain unusual postures, froth at the mouth, appear to be unaware of their surroundings, and talk in a strange voice. At such times, individuals who have grown up in the society believe that the shaman is possessed by a spirit. Afterwards, the shaman typically reports that he was possessed by a spirit, names the spirit that possessed him, and describes his experience of possession as different from his everyday experience. Despite the shaman's unusual behavior, the sincerity of his report, and the beliefs of other members of the culture, very few if any contemporary anthropologists would agree that the shaman was possessed by a spirit (Lewis, 1971). Why not? Certainly it is not because the shaman is simply lying or faking; there is every indication that he believes he was possessed by a spirit.

One reason for the anthropologist's skepticism is that the criteria for inferring the presence of spirit possession appear to be either ambiguous or circular. Another reason for skepticism stems from the anthropologist's belief that he can explain the shaman's behavior without utilizing the concept of *spirit possession*. For example, the anthropologist might contend that the shaman's behavior is role behavior; that is, it is behavior that is consistent with the shaman's own beliefs and expectations concerning what he is to experience, and it is also consistent with the beliefs and expectations of the other members of the community. The anthropologist might explain the shaman's report that he was possessed by a spirit by noting that the shaman's socialization led him to develop a set of beliefs and expectations consistent with the notion that certain experiences and behaviors are due to spirit possession. The shaman explains his experiences and behaviors in terms of spirit possession because this is the only term available in his culture for classifying them. Within the anthropologist's explanatory framework, however, an explanation in terms of spirit possession is unnecessary and unparsimonious.

Explanations of the shaman's behavior in terms of "spirit possession" are analogues to explanations of the hypnotic subject's behavior in terms of "hypnotic trance." Inferring the presence of "hypnotic trance" from the hypnotic subject's report that he was hypnotized or in a trance is about as misleading as inferring the presence of "spirit possession" from the shaman's report that he was possessed by a spirit. Just as we need not postulate "spirit possession" to explain the shaman's report, we need not postulate a special state of "hypnotic trance" to explain the hypnotic subject's report. The reports of both the shaman and the hypnotic subject can be adequately explained in terms of their beliefs and expectations. Let us look at how such an explanation would account for the reports given by some hypnotic subjects that they feel they are in a "hypnotic trance."

Typically, the subject in a hypnotic experiment is a student whose only acquaintance with hypnotism consists of what he has been exposed to in the popular media. Such an individual comes to the experimental setting with the following kinds of beliefs and expectations: (a) There is a special state or condition called a hypnotic state or hypnotic trance. (b) People are put in a hypnotic trance when they are exposed to a hypnotic induction procedure that tells them to become relaxed, drowsy, and sleepy. (c) While in a hypnotic trance, people have unusual experiences.

During the session, the "good" hypnotic subject finds that many of his beliefs and expectations about hypnotism are confirmed. He is told that he will be put into a hypnotic state or a hypnotic trance and he is then exposed to a "hypnotic induction procedure" stating that he is becoming relaxed, drowsy, and sleepy—"Your arms are relaxing . . . your body is relaxing . . . floating easily on a soft, cushiony cloud . . . becoming more and more relaxed . . . very relaxed and drowsy. . . ." This "good" subject thinks and imagines with the suggestions and, as he does so, he feels himself becoming relaxed and drowsy. He is then given a series of test suggestions that ask him to experience and do unusual things. For example, he may be told to clasp his hands together tightly and then given repeated suggestions that his hands are rigid, solid pieces of steel that are welded together. A feeling of rigidity is produced in the hands when the "good" subject clasps them tightly and contracts the muscles. As he then thinks and imagines with the suggestions, he focuses on the rigidity that is already present. In order to unclasp the rigid hands, it is necessary to remove the muscular contractions by relaxing the hands. However, the "good" subject does not relax the hands; instead, he continues to focus on the rigidity that is present and does not take them apart until he is told that he now can relax them. A little later he may be given the suggestion that one of his hands is "numb . . . dull . . . like a piece of rubber . . . insensitive." He may respond to this suggestion by thinking and imagining that his hand has been injected with Novocain and that it has become dull and insensitive, like a piece of rubber. To the extent that he thinks and imagines with the themes of the suggestion, he finds that the hand does feel numb and rubbery.

When later asked if he was hypnotized, this "good" hypnotic subject may answer "Yes." As in the case of the shaman who reports that he was possessed by a spirit, there is little reason to believe that the subject is simply lying. His experiences were generally congruent with his beliefs and expectations of what "being hypnotized" involves. He had experiences that he does not have in his day-to-day routine—not because it is so difficult to have the experiences but because situations are not found in daily life where a person is asked to think with the themes that are suggested and then is told repeatedly that he is becoming relaxed and drowsy or that his clasped hands are rigid or that other unusual effects are occurring. Similar to the case of the shaman, the subject's socialization has led him to believe that the variety of experiences that he had while responding to suggestions (for example, experiences of relaxation, drowsiness, hand rigidity, and numbness) are due to "being in hypnosis." Furthermore, since the subject was given only two major categories for classifying his experiences—as not hypnotized or as hypnotized to some degree—he is constrained from reporting his experiences in terms that fall outside of these two categories. For instance, he is constrained from reporting simply that he felt relaxed, drowsy, and ready and willing to respond to suggestions.

The foregoing considerations suggest three conclusions: (a) The reports given by some "good" hypnotic subjects—"I was hypnotized" or "I was in a hypnotic trance"—are in part a function of their beliefs and expectations concerning what "hypnosis" involves, interacting with the experiences they had while they were responding to suggestions. (b) Much more work is needed to sort out all of the complex interacting factors that determine whether a subject will state that he was or was not hypnotized. (c) The assertion that "A subject must be in a hypnotic trance because he says he is" is misleading in about the same way as the assertion that "A shaman must be possessed by a spirit because he says he is."

Believing one is hypnotized and responding to test suggestions. Before closing this section, it is appropriate to ask: If a subject believes that he is hypnotized, does this affect his responsiveness to test suggestions? Although it is questionable whether this belief *per se* directly affects the subject's responsiveness, it may affect his responsiveness in the following indirect way: If the subject responds to suggestions and judges from his responses that he is hypnotized, this might heighten his expectancy that he will respond to further suggestions, and the heightened expectancy may influence his subsequent response.

SUMMARY

This chapter focused on two questions:

1. *What variables in induction procedures give rise to a "hypnotic" appearance, changes in body feelings, and reports of having been hypnotized?*

The "hypnotic" appearance was shown to be due in part to keeping the eyes closed for a period of time (variable 4) and in part to suggestions for relaxation, sleep, and hypnosis (variable 5). Some of the changes in body feelings—for example, the experience of arm levitation or limb heaviness—were shown to be direct responses to the test suggestions. Other changes in body feelings—for example, changes in the size of the body or body parts and feelings of dizziness—were shown to be due in part to the subject expectantly focusing on and magnifying the feelings and sensations that are produced as he relaxes with his eyes closed while being told repeatedly that he is becoming relaxed, drowsy, sleepy, and is entering a hypnotic state. Subjects' reports that they were hypnotized were shown to be dependent upon (a) whether or not the hypnotist stated that they were hypnotized, (b) the wording of the questions that were submitted to them to elicit their reports, and (c) the degree of congruence between what they experienced and what they believe and expect that "hypnosis" involves.

2. *How do these three phenomena—"hypnotic" appearance, changes in body feelings, and reports of having been hypnotized—relate to responsiveness to test suggestions?* These phenomena have been traditionally viewed as indices of a "hypnotic trance"; in turn, the "hypnotic trance" has been regarded as a critical factor in producing heightened responsiveness to test suggestions. From our viewpoint, the three phenomena are not necessary, although two of the three—changes in body feelings and the subject believing that he is hypnotized—tend to be helpful in augmenting responsiveness to test suggestions. If a subject responds to the relaxation-sleep-hypnosis suggestions or to some of the other variables involved in induction procedures and, consequently, experiences changes in body feelings and judges from his responses that he is hypnotized, his expectancy that he can be affected by suggestions is enhanced. His enhanced expectancy, in turn, tends to heighten his responsiveness to subsequent test suggestions.

NOTES

[1] The control subjects were asked to open their eyes after five minutes had elapsed. Also they were recruited from a school in which no previous experiments had been conducted. They were told that they were participating in a psychological experiment and they accepted this definition of the situation—there was no indication that they defined the situation to themselves as hypnosis.

[2] Although we are discussing the factors that lead some subjects to state that they were hypnotized, it should be noted that many subjects who hypnotists judge to have been hypnotized do not believe that they were hypnotized. For instance, Wolberg (1972) writes: "One of the factors that complicates any definite interpretations of the nature of hypnosis is that most people after they have come out of [what the hypnotist judges as] a true hypnotic state believe that they were faking" (p. 48), and "Generally, the subject will deny having been in a hypnotic state, even when [according to the opinion of the hypnotist] he had achieved the deepest somnambulistic trance" (p. 49). Similarly, as we have pointed out elsewhere (Barber, 1969c), Milton H. Erickson typically judges about 65% of his subjects to have attained a "medium or deep trance" even though very few (about 17%) of his subjects believe that they were in a "medium or deep trance." In other words, it appears that hypnotists commonly believe that most of their subjects were hypnotized, whereas most of the subjects believe that they were not hypnotized.

[3] The Stanford Hypnotic Susceptibility Scales (Weitzenhoffer & Hilgard, 1959, 1962) include a standardized "hypnotic induction procedure," which focuses primarily on repeated suggestions of relaxation, drowsiness, and sleep, and a series of 12 standardized test suggestions. The test suggestions on these scales are similar to those included in the Barber Suggestibility Scale.

* * *

Gill and Brenman extract is from Gill, M.M. and Brenman, M. *Hypnosis and Related States*. New York: International Universities Press, Inc., 1959.

PART C

Mediating Variables

CHAPTER 5

Attitudes, Motivations, and Expectancies

From our cognitive-behavioral point of view, the extent to which subjects respond to test suggestions depends on their readiness to think and imagine with the themes that are suggested. Readiness, in turn, depends on attitudes, motivations, and expectancies (see Table 1, p. 20). In this chapter, we shall examine the role that attitudes, motivations, and expectancies play in affecting response to suggestions. In the next chapter, we turn our attention to the role of thinking and imagining with the themes that are suggested.

Attitudes, motivations, and expectancies toward being "hypnotized" or responding to suggestions each vary on a continuum from extremely positive to extremely negative. The positive end of each continuum can be described as follows:

Positive attitude. During the course of his life, the subject has acquired the view that being "hypnotized" or responding to suggestions is exciting, useful, worthwhile, or valuable.

Positive motivation. Right now, in the immediate test situation, the subject wants to be or tries to be "hypnotized" or to have the experiences that are suggested.

Positive expectancy. The subject believes that he himself can be "hypnotized" or can have the experiences that are suggested.

Although attitudes and motivations are usually highly correlated, they are at times separable. For instance, a subject may generally view "hypnosis" or responding to suggestions as worthwhile or valuable (positive attitude), but right now, in the specific situation with a specific experimenter, he does not want to be "hypnotized" or to respond to suggestions (negative motivation).

Furthermore, although attitudes and motivations are usually closely related to each other, they can both be clearly distinguished from expectancy. Even though a subject may generally view "hypnosis" or responding to suggestions as worthwhile and even though he may now try to be "hypnotized" or try to respond to the suggestions, he may *not* believe that he himself can be "hypnotized" or can have the experiences that are suggested.

Earlier investigators emphasized the importance of subjects' attitudes and motivations in determining their responsiveness to suggestions in a hypnotic situation. White (1941) noted that some subjects "who at first are insusceptible become excellent subjects when changes are made in the pattern of motives." Pattie (1956a) and Sarbin (1950a) also observed that some subjects were unresponsive to suggestions in one hypnotic session and very responsive in another session; they offered presumptive evidence that such changes were due to alteration in the subject's attitudes and motivations toward the test situation.

More recent investigations that pertain to the effects of attitudes, motivations, and expectancies can be divided into two sets. In one set of studies, an experimental attempt was made to alter the subjects' attitudes, motivations, or expectancies toward responding to suggestions or toward "hypnosis." In the other set of studies, the subjects were first asked to rate their attitudes, motivations, or expectancies toward "hypnosis" and then, after being exposed to a standardized induction procedure, were tested for responsiveness to test suggestions. We shall first summarize the studies that attempted to alter these factors experimentally and then we shall summarize the studies that used self-rating scales.

EXPERIMENTAL MANIPULATION OF ATTITUDES, MOTIVATIONS, AND EXPECTANCIES

A series of experimental studies indicate that attitudes, motivations, and expectancies play an important role in determining response to test suggestions.

Attempts to Produce Positive Motivations and Expectancies

In Chapter 3 of this text, experiments were cited in which subjects were exposed to a series of statements that were labeled *task motivational instructions*. Although this label emphasizes the motivational aspects of the instructions, a close look at the specific wording of the instructions indicates that they were aimed at producing not only positive motivation but also positive expectancies toward responding to test suggestions. The "task motivational instruc-tions" included statements that can be divided into two categories:

Statements in one category were intended to produce *positive motivation* (to desire and to try to have the experiences that are suggested):

> How well you do on the tests that I will give you depends entirely on your willingness to try to imagine and to visualize the things I will ask you to imagine. . . . What I ask is your cooperation in helping this experiment by trying to imagine vividly what I describe to you. . . . We're trying to measure the maximum ability of people to imagine. If you don't try to the best of your ability, this experiment will be worthless. . . .

Statements in the second category were intended to produce a *positive expectancy* on the part of the subject that he can have the experiences that are suggested:

> Everyone passed these tests when they tried. For example, we asked people to close their eyes and to imagine that they were at a movie theater and were watching a show. Most people were able to do this very well; they were able to imagine very vividly that they were at a movie and they felt as if they were actually looking at the picture. However, a few people thought that this was an awkward or silly thing to do and did not try to imagine and failed the test. Yet when these people later realized that it wasn't hard to imagine, they were able to visualize the movie picture and they felt as if the imagined movie was as vivid and as real as an actual movie. . . . If you try to imagine to the best of your ability, you can easily imagine and do the interesting things I tell you.

As stated in Chapter 3, these "task motivational instructions," which were intended to produce positive motivations and expectancies, raised responsiveness to the Barber Suggestibility Scale to about the same level found in a group exposed to a standardized "hypnotic induction procedure" and markedly above the level found in a control group. More precisely, 60% of the subjects who received the "task motivational instructions" showed a rather high level of response to the test suggestions (responding overtly to at least 5 of the 8 items on the Barber Suggestibility Scale and testifying that they experienced at least 5 of the suggested effects) as compared to 53% in the group exposed to repeated suggestions of relaxation, drowsiness, and sleep (the "hypnotic induction procedure") and 16% in the control group.

Attempts to Remove Negative Attitudes Toward "Hypnosis"

Several common misconceptions about "hypnosis" often give rise to negative attitudes. For instance, subjects often have the false belief that "hypnotized" subjects are under the control of the hypnotist and behave in a robot-like way. Consequently, they view "hypnosis" as something that should be resisted. Two experimental studies attempted to remove negative attitudes toward "hypnosis" by eliminating these kinds of misconceptions.

In one of these experiments (Cronin, Spanos, & Barber, 1971), half of the subjects were given favorable information about "hypnosis" that aimed to minimize negative attitudes by removing misconceptions. These subjects were told, for example, that

Hypnosis is not a state of semi-sleep in which individuals behave automatically in a mechanical and robot-like manner. . . . Subjects do not lose personal control of themselves. . . . In any hypnotic experiment it is the subject's cooperation that is necessary, rather than loss of control. No subject will be asked any questions of even remote personal content and no subject will be asked to do anything improper, [etc.]

The other half of the subjects were not told anything about hypnosis. Immediately afterwards, each subject was exposed to repeated suggestions of relaxation, drowsiness, and sleep and then was tested on the Barber Suggestibility Scale. As compared to the subjects who were not given any favorable information, those who had been given information intended to remove negative attitudes obtained significantly higher objective and subjective scores on the Barber Suggestibility Scale.

Diamond (1972) presented similar findings. Some of the subjects participating in Diamond's experiment were not given any preliminary information about hypnosis, while other subjects were given information that was designed to reduce negative attitudes by correcting misconceptions. The latter subjects, for instance, were told that they need not fear that they would lose control, that hypnosis is not mystical in any way, etc. Subjects who received information intended to minimize negative attitudes toward hypnosis scored significantly higher on the Stanford Hypnotic Susceptibility Scale than subjects who did not receive any information (cf. Gregory & Diamond, 1973).

Attempts to Produce Negative Attitudes and Motivations Toward Responding to Test Suggestions

Two experiments were designed to test the hypothesis that subjects with negative attitudes and motivations are unresponsive to test suggestions.

In the first experiment (Barber & Calverley, 1964e), subjects assigned to one group were told that they were to be tested for *gullibility* and then were individually tested immediately on the Barber Suggestibility Scale. Subjects randomly assigned to another group were told that they were to be tested for *ability to imagine* and then were tested individually on the same scale. A relatively high level of suggestibility (scores of 5 or above on the 8-point Barber Suggestibility Scale) was manifested by only 6% of the subjects who were told that they were being tested for gullibility as compared to 41% of the subjects who were told they were being tested for ability to imagine. Presumably, the statement to subjects that they were being tested for gullibility gave rise to a marked reduction in suggestibility by producing negative attitudes and motivations toward the test situation; that is, the subjects who were told that they were being tested for "gullibility" presumably did not view responding to suggestions as valuable and did not try to experience those things that were suggested.

In the second experiment (Barber & Calverley, 1964c), student nurses were tested on response to the Barber Suggestibility Scale immediately after they were exposed to one of the following three experimental treatments:

Treatment A (Task Motivational Instructions). These subjects were exposed to the task motivational instructions that were described previously in this chapter (p. 51).

Treatment B (Control). These subjects were simply told to try to imagine those things that would be suggested.

Treatment C (Attempt to Produce Negative Attitudes and Motivations). These subjects were told the following by their supervisor (the Supervisor of Student Nurses):

It's being rumored by doctors and administrators, and I don't know who else, that nursing students are too easily directed and easily led in their responses to suggestions. It's kind of shocking and discouraging to hear that the students are so easily directed and can't decide things for themselves. We've got a job to do—to impress the administrators and doctors around here with the fact that nursing students are not as gullible and as easily directed as they appear to have been showing during this research study. Well it sure is up to each of you as to how easily led, people around here think, student nurses are.

The three experimental treatments gave rise to markedly different scores on the Barber Suggestibility Scale. On the average, subjects under the Task Motivational treatment, the Control treatment, and the treatment in which an attempt was made to induce negative attitudes and motivations passed 4, 2, and 0, respectively, of the 8 test suggestions on the Barber Suggestibility Scale. In other words, when an attempt was made to produce negative attitudes and motivations toward responding to test suggestions, all subjects were nonsuggestible.

An attempt was also made in this experiment to determine what factors mediated the lack of suggestibility under Treatment C, in which an effort had been made to induce negative attitudes and motivations. The day after the experiment was completed, the subjects who had been tested under Treatment C were asked by the Supervisor of Student Nurses to write out the answer to the following question: "Did my statement to you yesterday about the experiment impress you in any way?" Answers to this question indicated that the failure of subjects assigned to Treatment C to be responsive to test suggestions was due to negative attitudes and motivations that were induced by the statement made by the Supervisor. For instance, a typical subject wrote: "I was impressed by the manner in which you expressed your concern over the project and the possible effect the outcome will have on the nursing profession. I agreed that we should have a mind of our own and should use it and that nurses should be firm in their decisions."

Attempts to Vary Expectancy

Three experiments that used different methods to influence subjects' expectancies indicate that expectancy plays an important role in determining responsiveness to test suggestions.

To produce a positive expectancy, Barber and Calverley (1964f) told half of the subjects, chosen at random, that it would be easy to respond to the suggestions they would be given. To produce a negative expectancy, the other half of the subjects were told that the suggestions were difficult to pass. Immediately afterwards, each subject was tested individually on the Barber Suggestibility Scale. Subjects given the instructions intended to produce a positive expectancy were significantly more responsive on the suggestibility scale than those given the instructions intended to produce a negative expectancy.

Klinger (1970) used the following strategy to vary subjects' expectancies: Before being tested on the Barber Suggestibility Scale, each subject observed another person (a stooge) responding to the scale. The stooge had been privately instructed to role-play a very suggestible person when he was observed by half of the subjects and to act as if he were very nonsuggestible when he was observed by the remaining subjects. Those subjects who saw the stooge responding without difficulty to the suggestions would presumably expect that it is easy to respond, while those who saw the stooge not responding to the suggestions would presumably expect that it is difficult to respond. Subjects who apparently had a more positive expectancy (who had observed the suggestible stooge) obtained an average score of 6.0 on the 8-point Barber Suggestibility Scale, whereas subjects who presumably had a negative expectancy (who had observed the unresponsive person) obtained an average score of 2.8 (cf. DeStefano, 1971; DeVoge & Sachs, 1971; Diamond, 1972; Marshall & Diamond, 1968).

To produce positive expectancies that the suggested effects can be experienced, Wilson (1967) asked half of the subjects to imagine various suggested effects while, without their knowledge, ingenious methods were used to help them experience each of the effects. For instance, each subject in this experimental group was asked to imagine that the room was red while a tiny bulb was secretly lit, providing a very faint tinge to the room. Immediately following these procedures, each subject in the experimental group was tested on the Barber Suggestibility Scale. The other half of the subjects, randomly assigned to a control condition, were not exposed to the secretly lit red bulb or to the other procedures that might lead them to expect that they could experience suggested effects. Instead, the control subjects were simply tested on the Barber Suggestibility Scale. Subjects in the experimental group obtained an average score of 5, whereas those in the control group obtained a significantly lower average score of 3 on the 8-point Barber Suggestibility Scale.

SELF-RATINGS OF ATTITUDES, MOTIVATIONS, AND EXPECTANCIES

Let us now summarize a series of studies that used self-rating scales to measure attitudes, motivations, or expectancies toward "hypnosis."

Attitudes

A series of studies used various types of scales to measure subjects' attitudes toward "hypnosis" and used either the Stanford Hypnotic Susceptibility Scale or the Barber Suggestibility Scale to assess subjects' responsiveness to test suggestions in a hypnotic situation. Two studies (Andersen, 1963; Melei & Hilgard, 1964) found small to moderate positive correlations—for example, a correlation of .47 (Andersen, 1963) between attitudes to "hypnosis" and responsiveness to test suggestions.[1] A subsequent study (Barber & Calverley, 1966c) yielded a correlation of .55 between one type of attitude measure (perceiving hypnosis as interesting) and objective scores on the Barber Suggestibility Scale. Another study (Diamond, Gregory, Lenney, Steadman, & Talone, 1972) yielded a correlation of .47 between another type of attitude measure (perceiving hypnosis as desirable) and scores on the Stanford Hypnotic Susceptibility Scale.

Motivation

Motivation to be hypnotized was assessed by Calverley and Barber (unpublished data) using a scale that asked the subject whether he wanted to be hypnotized and, if so, whether he wanted to be hypnotized to a deep, medium, or light level. Scores on this scale were positively correlated (r = .36) with scores on the Stanford Hypnotic Susceptibility Scale. Similarly, J. R. Hilgard (1970) obtained a small but significant correlation (.25) between motivation for hypnosis and scores on the Stanford scale.

Expectancies

A series of studies used various types of scales to measure subjects' expectations of their own hypnotizability and either the Stanford scale or the Barber scale to assess responsiveness to test suggestions in a hypnotic situation. Melei and Hilgard (1964) and also Dermen and London (1965) found small positive correlations between subjects' expectations of their own hypnotizability and their scores on a hypnotic susceptibility scale. Other studies (Barber & Calverley, 1966c, 1969; Gregory & Diamond, 1973; Unestahl, 1969) obtained significant correlations, ranging from .33 to .62 between subjects' preexperimental expectations of their own hypnotizability and their responses to suggestions in a hypnotic situation.

Another series of studies (London, Cooper, & Johnson, 1962; Rosenhan & Tomkins, 1964; Shor, 1971; Shor, Orne, & O'Connell, 1966) generally yielded positive correlations (which were more often significant for females than for males) between response to test suggestions in a hypnotic situation and either preexperimental *attitudes* toward hypnosis or preexperimental *expectations* of hypnotizability.[2]

SUMMARY

Two sets of studies have been reviewed in this chapter. The first set attempted to manipulate attitudes, motivations, or expectancies experimentally. These studies indicated that (a) after an attempt is made to produce positive motivations and expectancies toward responding to suggestions, 60% of the subjects show a relatively high level of response to test suggestions (as compared to 16% in a control group), (b) after an attempt is made to remove negative attitudes toward "hypnosis," subjects obtain higher scores on the Barber Suggestibility Scale or the Stanford Hypnotic Susceptibility Scale, (c) after an attempt is made to produce negative attitudes and motivations toward the test situation, subjects show little or no responsiveness to test suggestions, and (d) after an attempt is made to induce positive expectancies in one group and negative expectancies in another, the scores of the "positive expectancy" group on the 8-point Barber Suggestibility Scale are generally 2 or 3 points higher than the scores of the "negative expectancy" group.

In the second set of studies, attitudes, motivations, or expectancies toward "hypnosis" were assessed on rating scales that were completed by the subjects before they participated in the experiment. These studies found positive correlations (typically in the range of .30 to .50) between subject's preexperimental attitudes, motivations, or expectancies and their responsiveness to test suggestions in a hypnotic situation.

These data appear to justify two conclusions: (a) attitudes, motivations, and expectancies play a role in determining responsiveness to test suggestions and (b) further research is needed to develop more effective methods of enhancing subjects' attitudes, motivations, and expectancies toward the test situation.

NOTES .

[1] Correlations express the degree of relationship between two variables. Correlations around .30 indicate that there is a very small relationship between the variables, correlations around .50 or .60 indicate a moderate relationship, and correlations of .70 or higher indicate that there is a substantial relationship between the variables.

[2] A problem inherent in all of the studies that used self-rating scales, and in some of the studies that attempted to manipulate attitudes, motivations, and expectancies experimentally, is that they measured or attempted to vary attitudes, motivations, or expectancies toward a term—"hypnosis"—that is loaded with surplus meaning. The term "hypnosis" has a wide variety of connotations and subjects have all sorts of misconceptions about what a "hypnosis" session actually involves. Also, with few exceptions, the subjects participating in these studies had not previously participated in a hypnotic experiment. Soon after the hypnotic session had begun, the subjects may have seen that "hypnosis" is quite different from what they thought it would be and may have changed their attitudes, motivations, or expectancies. Consequently, further studies in this area should also try to assess changes in subjects' attitudes, motivations, and expectancies during the course of the hypnotic session. We might predict that higher correlations between attitudes, motivations, and expectancies and responses to test suggestions will be obtained when the former variables are measured after the subject has had a chance to see what "hypnosis" actually involves.

CHAPTER 6

Thinking and Imagining with the Themes of the Suggestions

A basic postulate that underlies this text is that subjects are responsive to test suggestions when they think and imagine with the themes that are suggested. This postulate is generally harmonious with the viewpoint of Sarbin and his associates (Juhasz, 1969; Sarbin, 1950, 1972; Sarbin & Coe, 1972; Sarbin & Juhasz, 1970) who have focused on the concept of imagining. These investigators have criticized earlier conceptualizations that viewed imaginings as "conditioned sensations" or as quasi-perceptual "pictures in the mind." As an alternative, Sarbin and his coworkers have suggested that imagining can be more fruitfully conceptualized as an active process that is more similar to muted, attenuated, role-taking rather than to a passive "looking at" quasi-objects in a hypothetical mind-space. For these investigators, imagining is "an active form of conduct, a performance, a doing, that had its origins in the practice of imitating with models present and of imitating with models absent" (Sarbin, 1972, p. 344). Also, Sarbin and his coworkers view imagining as involving a large component of "as if" behavior. When an individual is imagining, he is to some extent acting *as if* certain hypothetical events are in fact occurring. These investigators have also argued that imagining can be usefully conceptualized as falling along a dimension of involvement where the degree of involvement refers to the intensity with which the process is carried out. Sarbin and Coe (1972) have further pointed out that the tendency to become involved in imagining can be conceptualized as a skill possessed by individuals to different degrees. Successful enactment of the hypnotic role calls for one aspect of this skill—namely, the ability to become involved in imaginings that are generated by verbal suggestions.

How does this process of imagining lead to the overt behaviors and the subjective experiences that have been historically associated with the term

59

"hypnotism"? An important but neglected paper by Arnold (1946) provides some preliminary answers to this question.

First, Arnold points out that "words may be considered as symbols which stand for the situation or activity they refer to." When we hear words that describe a previous experience, the experience tends to be reinstated in a sketchy, fragmentary way; we tend to visualize or feel ourselves in the previous situation and we tend to reexperience the attitudes and reactions that were present in that situation. When the experimenter repeatedly suggests to the subject that his arm feels heavy or very light or numb, he is inviting the subject to imagine vividly previous situations in which he had these experiences and, as a result of the vivid imagining, to reinstate the attitudes, feelings, and reactions that he had previously experienced.

Secondly, Arnold summarizes a series of studies that indicated that thinking about and imagining a suggested movement or activity tends to bring about that movement or activity. Arnold refers to the well-known experiments of Jacobson (1930, 1932), which showed that an imagined movement (for example, bending one arm) is associated with small but measurable contractions in the flexor muscles of the arm. If the subject is relaxed when he is imagining the movement, minimal muscular contractions always occur in the limb that is imagined as moving and they do not occur in the other limbs or the trunk. Extending Jacobson's preliminary results, Arnold (1946) and Schultz (1932) showed that whenever a subject is simply told to imagine that he is falling forward or backward, he moves in the imagined direction to some extent. In addition to asking the subject to imagine falling forward or backward, several investigators (Arnold, 1946; Hull, 1933; Mordey, 1960; Schultz, 1932) also asked subjects to think or to imagine that one of their arms was moving up or down, or that a pendulum (which they held by two fingers on one hand) was moving to the right or left. The subjects tended to show movement in the suggested direction and those who reported imagining the most vividly showed the most marked movement in the specified direction. In general, subjects who did not manifest the suggested movement stated afterwards that they did not imagine or that they thought of something else.

Thirdly, Arnold summarizes studies that show that imagining an event sometimes produces physiological changes that are found when the event actually occurs. For instance, Schultz (1926) asked subjects who had been trained to relax thoroughly to imagine vividly that their forehead was cool. Temperature measurements showed that in about one-third of the subjects the forehead became cool while they were imagining it. Presumably, the drop in the temperature of the forehead was produced by a contraction of the superficial blood vessels (vasoconstriction). Conversely, Schultz found that relaxed subjects who were asked to imagine vividly that their hand was exposed to heat tended to experience a sensation of warmth which was associated in about 80% of the subjects with a rise in skin temperature up to about 2° C.

Other investigators have presented similar results. For instance, Hadfield (1920) and Menzies (1941) found that some individuals show vasoconstriction and a drop in the temperature of the skin when they are instructed to think about and to imagine that a limb is cold; conversely, they show vasodilation and a rise in the temperature of the skin when asked to think about and to imagine that a limb is warm. Similarly, Harano, Ogawa, and Naruse (1965) asked subjects to repeat to themselves and to focus on the idea, "My arms are warm." When thinking and imagining on this theme, subjects generally exhibited several interrelated changes in the arms—a change in experienced warmth, an increase in the surface temperature, and an increase in blood volume. It is important to note that Harano et al. did *not* find these changes in the arms when the subjects tried purposively to raise the temperature of the arms without thinking or imagining that the arms were warm.

In brief, a series of investigations indicate that (a) thinking about and imagining movements (of the limbs, body, etc.) tend to bring about the actual movements, (b) thinking about and imagining an event, such as "My arm is warm," tend to give rise to physiological changes that are found when the event actually occurs, and (c) in broader terms, thinking and imagining with the themes that are suggested tend to produce both the overt behaviors and subjective experiences that are suggested. Let us now turn to three recent studies (Spanos, 1971; Spanos & Barber, 1972; Spanos & Ham, 1973) that extended these results by focusing on a specific kind of imagining—*goal-directed imagining*.

GOAL-DIRECTED IMAGINING

The first experiment (Spanos, 1971) aimed to probe more intensively into the relationship between imagining and responding to test suggestions. The subjects were 24 female nursing students. At the beginning of each experimental session, each subject was told individually:

I am interested in what is going on in people's minds when they are hypnotized. I'm interested in what they are thinking, imagining, feeling, and saying to themselves during hypnosis. In this experiment I am going to hypnotize you and ask you to carry out some suggestions. After each suggestion, while you are still hypnotized, I'll ask you to tell me what was passing through your mind while you were carrying out the suggestion. In giving me your answer, it's very important that you be honest and tell me everything that was passing through your mind— everything that you were thinking, imagining, feeling, and saying to yourself—even if you think it silly or unimportant.

Repeated suggestions of relaxation, sleep, and hypnosis were administered and then the subject was given a series of standardized test suggestions for arm heaviness, arm levitation, rigidity of the hands, selective amnesia, etc. Immediately after completing each test suggestion, the subject was asked to report what was passing through her mind during the time she was receiving the suggestion. In about 80% of the cases, the subjects who passed a specific test suggestion reported that they were imagining in a specific way; namely, *they were imagining a situation which, if it actually occurred, would tend to give rise to the behavior that was suggested.* Typical examples of this type of imagining, which Spanos labeled *goal-directed fantasy* or *imagining*, were as follows: A subject who passed a test suggestion that her arm was light and was rising reported: "I imagined that my arm was hollow, there was nothing in it, and somebody was putting air into it." A subject who passed a test suggestion for arm heaviness reported: "I imagined that there were all kinds of rocks tied to my arm. It felt heavy and I could feel it going down."

An important finding in the experiment was that subjects who passed the test suggestions at times disregarded the specific things they were told to imagine. Instead, they imagined something different that would also tend to give rise to the suggested overt behavior. For instance, a subject who was told that she would not be able to say her name because she would "Imagine that the muscles in your throat and jaw are solid and rigid, as if they're made of steel . . ." reported imagining instead that "Somebody had their hands around my neck. . . . It was a man whose hands were big and hairy and dirty." Reports of this type indicated that the responsive subjects did not necessarily regard the specific contents of the suggestions as directives that they had to follow in detail. Instead, they tended to view the contents of the suggestions as guides for goal-directed imagining—that is, as guides for imagining situations which, if they actually transpired, would tend to give rise to the suggested behavior.[1]

In a second experiment (Spanos & Ham, 1973), a suggestion for selective amnesia (to forget the number 4) was given to a group that had been exposed to repeated suggestions of relaxation, drowsiness, sleep, and hypnosis and to a control group that had not been exposed to such suggestions. With few exceptions, subjects in both groups who appeared to manifest selective amnesia (who did not verbalize the number 4) reported goal-directed imagining. For instance, one subject imagined the numbers 1 through 5 on a blackboard and then imagined that the number 4 had been erased; another subject imagined the numbers 1 through 10 and then imagined that the number 4 "was sort of going into the distance like a rocket ship would go into space and then, finally, it was gone."

In a third experiment (Spanos & Barber, 1972), subjects were exposed to repeated suggestions of relaxation, drowsiness, sleep, and hypnosis and then were given suggestions for arm levitation. Each subject was then asked to report what was passing through his mind when he was given the suggestion for arm levitation. The subjects' reports were scored for the presence or absence of goal-directed imagining.[2] Subsequently, each subject who had passed the test suggestion completed a rating scale that asked to what extent the arm levitation was experienced as involuntary ("I experienced the arm rising completely by itself"), partially involuntary, or totally voluntary ("I only had the experience of causing the arm to rise"). Goal-directed imagining and the experience of involuntariness were related as follows: (a) *All* of the subjects who carried out goal-directed imagining—who imagined a situation which, if it had actually occurred, would result in the arm moving up—felt that the arm levitation occurred involuntarily. (b) Of those who did not carry out goal-directed imagining, only 40% felt that the arm levitation occurred involuntarily.

It is important at this point to emphasize again that the *wording of suggestions* plays an important role in determining the subjects' experiences. We noted above that subjects often define their overt response to a suggestion as an involuntary occurrence. However, it is the wording of the test suggestions that (a) informs the subjects that it is appropriate to define their responses as involuntary and (b) provides them with a strategy for defining their behavior in this way. The kinds of suggestions used in hypnotic experiments do not ask the subjects to carry out overt acts voluntarily. Instead, they usually provide the subjects with a strategy for defining their behavior as involuntary by asking them to imagine situations which, if they were to occur in reality, would tend to produce the desired behavior. For example, the behavioral criterion for passing the arm heaviness suggestion of the Stanford Hypnotic Susceptibility Scale (Form C) consists of the subject lowering his outstretched arm (Weitzenhoffer & Hilgard, 1962). This suggestion does not directly instruct the subject to lower his arm. Instead, the suggestion is worded as follows: ". . . Imagine you are holding something heavy in your hand. . . . Now the hand and arm feel heavy as if the [imagined] weight were pressing down . . . and as it feels heavier and heavier the hand and arm begin to move down. . . ." If the situation described by this suggestion were to occur objectively (if the subject were to actually hold a weight in his hand), then his arm would become heavy and would tend to move downward, and he would attribute the heaviness and lowering to the presence of the weight rather than to a volitional act.

Many other test suggestions used in hypnotic experiments also provide subjects with a cognitive strategy by instructing them to engage in specific patterns of imagining: "I want you to imagine a force acting on your hands to push them apart . . ." (Weitzenhoffer & Hilgard, 1962). "Imagine your hands are two pieces of steel that are welded together so that it is impossible to get them apart . . ." (Barber, 1965a). "Think of your arm becoming stiffer and stiffer . . . as if it were in a splint so the elbow cannot bend . . ." (Weitzenhoffer & Hilgard, 1962). Each of these test suggestions clearly instructs the subject to engage in goal-directed imagining.

SUMMARY

The data presented in this chapter indicate the following (a) Thinking and imagining with the themes that are suggested tend to produce both the overt behaviors and the subjective experiences that are suggested. (b) Subjects who pass test suggestions commonly report that they engaged in goal-directed imagining—that is, they imagined situations which, if they occurred in reality, would tend to produce the suggested behavior. (c) Goal-directed imagining provides the subject with a strategy for defining his overt acts as involuntary occurrences. (d) Test suggestions commonly instruct the subject to engage in goal-directed imagining.

NOTES

[1] Subjects in the experiment who did not pass a test suggestion either reported that (a) they were unwilling to cooperate or to respond to the suggestion (e.g., "I was kind of hoping that I would be able to pull my hands apart") or (b) they tried to cooperate but they did not imagine. An illustrative report that falls into the latter category (a subject who tried to cooperate but did not imagine) was as follows: "When you said that my hands would be stuck together, I tried to make them so. I held them tight and pushed hard . . . but it just didn't work."

[2] These judgments could be made reliably by two raters who agreed in every instance. For instance, it was clear that the following report should be scored as goal-directed imagining: "I imagined a balloon tied to my arm and the balloon was slowly rising."

PART D

The Wonders of Hypnotism

CHAPTER 7

Perceptual and Physiological Effects, Age Regression, Visual Hallucinations, and Trance Logic

For nearly 200 years, a wide variety of extraordinary phenomena have been associated with hypnotism. These "marvels" include the following: (a) the production of perceptual effects such as deafness, blindness, and colorblindness, (b) the elicitation of physiological changes such as the cure of warts, (c) the reinstatement of childhood behaviors and experiences by hypnotic age regression, (d) the production of visual hallucinations, (e) the elicitation of unusual cognitive processes such as trance logic, (f) the production of surgical anesthesia, and (g) the elicitation of extraordinary feats in stage hypnotism. At first glance, these kinds of phenomena might seem to be more easily explained by the "hypnotic trance" viewpoint rather than by our cognitive-behavioral viewpoint. Let us see if this is actually the case. The first five phenomena listed above will be discussed in this chapter and the last two phenomena—surgical anesthesia and stage hypnotism—will be discussed in Chapters 8 and 9.

PERCEPTUAL EFFECTS (DEAFNESS, BLINDNESS, AND COLORBLINDNESS)

A few researchers have seriously contended that "hypnotized" subjects actually become deaf when they are given suggestions of deafness. For instance, Erickson (1938) reported that 6 of 30 selected subjects, who were given suggestions of deafness when they were judged to be in "hypnotic trance," did not react to unexpected sounds, did not raise their voice to overcome a disturbing extraneous noise, and did not respond to deliberately embarrassing remarks. From these and similar data, Erickson concluded that "there was produced a condition not distinguishable from neurological deafness by any of the ordinarily competent tests employed."

Erickson's conclusion does not follow from the data he presented. For instance, failure to react to unexpected sounds does not demonstrate that the sounds were not heard. In an earlier experiment (Dynes, 1932), three selected "hypnotized" subjects, who had received suggestions of deafness, did not show any reaction when a pistol was fired unexpectedly. However, each of these subjects testified postexperimentally that he had clearly heard the pistol shot. Similarly, failure to raise one's voice when there is a disturbing noise and failure to respond to deliberately embarrassing remarks do not demonstrate that the subject cannot hear because these responses can be rather easily inhibited voluntarily.

To determine the effects of suggested deafness, we (Barber & Calverley, 1964d) and other investigators (Kline, Guze & Haggerty, 1954; Kramer & Tucker, 1967; Scheibe, Gray, & Keim, 1968; Sutcliffe, 1961) used a sensitive method that is called *delayed auditory feedback*. Let us explain how this method works.

Auditory feedback is a procedure whereby a person wearing earphones speaks and hears his own voice played back to him through the earphones. In delayed auditory feedback, the individual's voice is not played back the instant that he speaks. Instead, his voice is delayed a fraction of a second so that he hears not what he is saying but what he has just said. When an individual with normal hearing is exposed to delayed auditory feedback, he typically begins to talk more slowly, to mispronounce words, and to stumble over his words. However, the speech of deaf individuals is not affected by delayed auditory feedback.

In our experiment (Barber & Calverley, 1964d), suggestions of deafness were given to hypnotic subjects—that is, to subjects who had been exposed to a standardized hypnotic induction procedure that focused on relaxation-sleep-hypnosis suggestions. Suggestions of deafness were also given to control subjects who had *not* been exposed to a hypnotic induction procedure. All subjects were then tested for response to delayed auditory feedback. None of the subjects, even those who insisted that they could not hear, behaved like individuals who are actually deaf. That is, both the hypnotic subjects and the control subjects responded to the delayed auditory feedback with slowing of speech, mispronunciations of words, and stammering. These results, together with those presented by other investigators (Kline et al., 1954; Kramer & Tucker, 1967; Scheibe et al.,

1968; Sutcliffe, 1961), clearly indicated that hypnotic subjects who are supposedly deaf are able to hear.

Although the "hypnotic deaf" subject may be trying not to hear, he simply does not succeed in completely blocking out sounds. The fact that the subject can hear is sometimes rather obvious. For instance, after deafness has been suggested, the experimenter may ask, "Can you hear me?" A few "hypnotized" subjects will answer, "No, I can't hear you." The remaining subjects who do not respond to the question may appear to be deaf. However, these subjects can be brought out of their "hypnotic deafness" if the experimenter states: "Now you can hear again." Since the subjects now respond to auditory stimulation, it is obvious that they could hear all along.

Similar considerations apply to "hypnotic blindness." If "hypnotized" subjects are told that they are blind, they typically try not to see—they may cross their eyes, stare at one point in space, or unfocus their eyes. Although they try not to see, they are not blind (Barber, 1970). In fact, the "hypnotized" subject who is given suggestions of blindness typically does what you or I would also do if we were in an experimental situation and we were motivated to respond to suggestions. If given suggestions of blindness, we would try to the best of our ability not to see, we might try to blur our vision or to stare at one spot, but we would not succeed in becoming blind.

Erickson (1939) also claimed that suggestions given to subjects in "hypnotic trance" can produce colorblindness. Colorblindness is typically assessed by showing subjects a series of cards comprised of many colored dots. The dots are arranged in such a way that a person with normal color vision perceives certain numbers and letters on the cards whereas a colorblind person perceives a different set of numbers and letters. Erickson administered one of these tests, the Ishihara Test for Colorblindness, to hypnotic subjects who had been given suggestions of colorblindness. The subjects typically reported the same numbers that are reported by colorblind individuals, and Erickson concluded that hypnotically induced colorblindness is indistinguishable from actual colorblindness. However, Erickson failed to ascertain whether control subjects who are simply asked to ignore certain colors might also respond in the same way to the Ishihara cards. To test this possibility, we gave a test for colorblindness to control subjects who were told to try their best to ignore the colors for which Erickson had suggested blindness (Barber & Deeley, 1961). The control subjects also typically behaved like colorblind individuals. These findings suggest that Erickson's hypnotic subjects may not have experienced colorblindness but may instead have simply tried to ignore some of the colors that they were looking at.

PHYSIOLOGICAL EFFECTS

Experimental studies indicate that suggestions given to subjects who are in a "hypnotic trance" are at times effective in (a) producing acceleration and also deceleration of the heart (Klemme, 1963), (b) improving visual acuity in near-sighted individuals (Graham & Leibowitz, 1972; Harwood, 1971; Kelley, 1958, 1961), (c) inhibiting allergic responses (Ikemi & Nakagawa, 1962), (d) inhibiting gastric hunger contractions and increasing stomach acid secretions (Ikemi, 1959; Lewis & Sarbin, 1943; Luckhardt & Johnston, 1924), (e) curing warts (Sinclair-Gieben & Chalmers, 1959; Surman, Gottlieb, Hackett, & Silverberg, 1973; Ullman & Dudek, 1960), and (f) producing various other physiological alterations (Barber, 1961c, 1965b, 1970; McPeake, 1968; Sarbin, 1956; Sarbin & Slagle, 1972). We can view these kinds of effects in perspective by noting the following:

In general, when the experiments included control subjects who received the same suggestions as the "hypnotized" subjects, about the same number of both kinds of subjects showed the suggested effects (Barber, 1961c, 1965b, 1970; McPeake, 1968). For instance, suggestions that the heart was accelerating and also suggestions that it was decelerating were as effective with control subjects as with subjects who were said to be in "hypnotic trance" in producing the suggested change in heart rate (Klemme, 1963). Also, suggestions intended to improve nearsighted vision were effective with control subjects and with "hyp-notized" subjects in producing a change in visual acuity (Graham & Leibowitz, 1972; Harwood, 1971, Kelley, 1958, 1961).

Similarly, suggestions intended to inhibit allergic responses were as effective with control subjects as with "hypnotized" subjects in reducing the allergic responses (Ikemi & Nakagawa, 1962). Along the same lines, although suggestions of eating a delicious meal are at times effective in increasing stomach secretions in some subjects who are said to be in "hypnotic trance," some individuals show similar effects in ordinary life situations when they think about or vividly imagine delicious foods (Luckhardt & Johnston, 1924; Miller, Bergeim, Rehfuss, & Hawk, 1920; Wolf & Wolff, 1947). The same considerations apply to the cure of warts: although suggestions for wart removal are apparently effective at times when they are given to "hypnotized" subjects, they also appear to be effective at times when they are given to control subjects (Allington, 1934; Bloch, 1927; Bonjour, 1929; Dudek, 1967; Sulzberger & Wolf, 1934; Vollmer, 1946).[1] In brief, although much more work is needed to clarify how suggestions affect body processes, the data available at present do not support the notion that "hypnotic trance" is a critical factor in producing such physiological effects.[2]

AGE REGRESSION

Age regression has long been considered to be one of the most dramatic aspects of hypnotism. For instance, it has been reported that, when subjects in "hypnotic trance" are given suggestions for age regression, they behave just like four-month-old infants (Gidro-Frank & Bowersbuch, 1948) or they recall the exact day of the week on which their birthdate fell when they were children (True, 1949). Since such special effects were produced, one might contend that the subjects were in a "special state" and were not simply thinking about and vividly imagining an earlier time. Let us look in turn at the studies by Gidro-Frank and Bowersbuch and by True that seem to contradict our viewpoint and to support the "hypnotic trance" viewpoint.

Babinski Reflex During Hypnotic Regression to Infancy

Gidro-Frank and Bowersbuch (1948) suggested to six selected subjects in "deep trance" that they were four months of age. Why did these investigators choose the age of four months? Because textbooks stated that, when the four-month-old infant is stimulated on the sole of the foot, he shows a Babinski reflex—his large toe moves backward and his other toes spread out. Textbooks also stated that at six months of age or older individuals show the normal response in which the toes move forward. Thus, Gidro-Frank and Bowersbuch tried to determine whether "hypnotic regression" to four months of age reinstates a physiological response (the Babinski reflex) that is characteristic of the four-month-old infant. They reported that three of the six selected subjects "went back" psychophysiologically to the age of four months—they showed the Babinski response.

This experiment seemed to support the contention that, since responsive hypnotic subjects can show a special reflex, they must be in a special state. However, this contention is invalid because the experiment was based on fallacy. Textbooks that stated that four-month-old infants show a Babinski response were misleading—four-month-old infants are *not* characterized by a Babinski response. Burr (1921) noted such wide variations in the response of 69 infants as to conclude that no specific movements of the toes could be considered as characteristic of the infantile response to stimulation on the sole of the foot. Similarly, Wolff (1930) observed an unequivocal Babinski response in only 13 of 389 observations made on infants below seven months of age. In brief, the Babinski response is *not* a characteristic response of infants. It appears that textbook writers copied their wrong statements from one another without bothering to observe infants closely.

There are several possible reasons why three of the six adult subjects in the Gidro-Frank and Bowersbuch experiment showed a Babinski response (Barber, 1969b, 1970). For instance, the subjects may have become aware of the purpose of the experiment and may have voluntarily performed the Babinski response; that is, they may have purposively moved their large toe backwards while spreading out the other toes (Sarbin, 1956). However, the reasons why three of the six adult subjects showed a Babinski response are not especially important. What is important is that the Gidro-Frank and Bowersbuch experiment did not demonstrate a special effect that is unique to four-month-old infants; consequently, it is inappropriate to argue from the results of the experiment that the subjects must have been in a special state.

Exact Recall of Past Birthdays

A study by True (1949) seemed to indicate that "hypnotized" subjects who are given suggestions for age regression show a marvelous ability to recall events that had occurred during childhood. In this study, the subjects were exposed to an induction procedure and were then given suggestions that they were 11 years of age, 7 years of age, and 4 years of age. At each of the "regressed" ages, the subjects were told that it was their birthday or Christmas day and they were asked to name the day of the week. In the great majority of instances (81% of the time), the subjects named the correct day of the week on which their birthday or Christmas day fell when they were 11, 7, and 4 years of age. One might conclude from these results that, since the hypnotic subjects were able to recall earlier dates in a very special way, they must have been in a very special state.

However, eight subsequent investigations failed to confirm True's results (Barber, 1961b; Best & Michaels, 1954; Cooper & Morgan, 1966; Fisher, 1962; Leonard, 1963; Mesel & Ledford, 1959; O'Connell, Shor, & Orne, 1970; Reiff & Scheerer, 1959). Why did True obtain different results from the other eight sets of investigators? O'Connell, Shor, and Orne (1970) have pointed out that (a) True was aware of the actual day of the week upon which each former birthday or Christmas day fell, (b) True asked each subject in progression, "Was it Sunday? Was it Monday? Was it Tuesday?" and (c) his tone and inflections when asking the questions may have provided the subjects with the correct answer. Another possibility is that the subjects told each other the formula for computing previous dates; this involves the simple principle that the days of the week go backward one day each year and two on leap years (Barber, 1962a; Sutcliffe, 1960; Yates, 1960). Although we cannot say with certainty why True obtained results that differed from those obtained in eight subsequent, carefully conducted investigations, the important point is that until True's results are replicated they cannot be interpreted as supporting the "hypnotic trance" viewpoint.[3]

A Perspective Toward "Hypnotic Age Regression"

We believe our cognitive-behavioral viewpoint is consistent with the experimental data pertaining to "hypnotic age regression." Let us first summarize the experimental findings and then see how they are harmonious with our viewpoint.

Empirical studies in this area indicate the following:

1. When subjects who are said to be in "hypnotic trance" are given suggestions that they are children, they tend to perform somewhat like children (on intelligence tests, on the Rorschach, on the Bender-Gestalt, on drawing tests, etc.). However, their performance is generally at a level that is somewhat superior to the norms for the specified age or to the subject's own original performance at the earlier age (Crasilneck & Michael, 1957; Hoskovec & Horvai, 1963; Leonard, 1965; O'Connell, Shor, & Orne, 1970; Orne, 1951; Sarbin, 1950b; Sarbin & Farberow, 1952; Taylor, 1950; Troffer, 1966; Young, 1940).

2. The childlike performance that is produced by "hypnotic age regression" can also be produced by instructing either a control subject or a "hypnotized" subject to play the role of a child or to simulate a child's performance (Gordon & Freston, 1964; Greenleaf, 1969; Hoskovec & Horvai, 1963; O'Connell, Shor, & Orne, 1970; Solomon & Goodson, 1971; Staples & Wilensky, 1968; Troffer, 1966).

3. When subjects are randomly assigned to a hypnotic induction group and to a control group, and subjects in both groups are given suggestions to go back or to regress to an earlier time, the same proportion of subjects in both groups testify that they imagined, felt, or believed that they had returned to the earlier time (Barber & Calverley, 1966a).

4. Subjects who give a childlike performance when "hypnotically regressed" to childhood also give an equally convincing portrayal of an older individual or of a senile individual when "hypnotically progressed" to the age of 70, 80, or 90 (Kline, 1951; Rubenstein & Newman, 1954).

In the light of the foregoing, we would conceptualize the data pertaining to "age regression" as follows: (a) When hypnotic subjects or control subjects are told to "regress" to a past time in their lives, most of the subjects try and some succeed in thinking and imagining that they are in the past. (b) Those who succeed in vividly imagining the past, or who become "involved" in imagining, tend to feel as if, and to a certain extent behave as if, they are in a past time. The phenomenon of "hypnotic age progression" can also be viewed in the same way; that is, when given suggestions to "progress" to the future, some subjects succeed in vividly imagining a future time and to a certain extent feel as if they are in a future time.

VISUAL HALLUCINATIONS

Most texts on hypnotism state that visual hallucinations can be produced by appropriate suggestions given to hypnotic subjects. For instance, Estabrooks (1943) states:

> We proceed somewhat as follows: "Listen carefully. When I give the word you will open your eyes but you will not wake up. . . . You will see standing on the table in front of you a very friendly black cat. You will go over, pet the cat, then lift it up carefully and put it on the chair in which you have been seated" . . . The subject must be in a deep somnambulism if he is to be subject to these hallucinations. . . . Should he really have a vision of the cat, his actions will be characteristic. He will pet the animal and play with it in so convincing a fashion that the operator need have no doubt as to what has really happened. [p. 20-21].

Accounts of this type strongly imply that "hypnotized" subjects do not simply vividly visualize or imagine the suggested object. On the contrary, they imply that subjects who are in a "deep somnambulistic trance" actually *see* a suggested object in the same way that they *see* an actual object. Recent research indicates that these implications are misleading.

A series of studies (Barber & Calverley, 1964a; Bowers, 1967; McPeake & Spanos, 1973; Spanos & Barber, 1968; Spanos, Ham, & Barber, 1973) indicates that whether subjects state that they *imagined* or *saw* the suggested object is markedly affected by the *wording* of the questions that ask them to describe their experiences. In these studies, the subjects were asked to rate the vividness and reality of the suggested hallucination on either one of two kinds of rating scales. One of the rating scales did *not* permit the subject to report that he had *imagined* the suggested object—that is, it included only the categories *did not see it*, *vaguely saw it*, *clearly saw it*, and *saw it and believed it was there*. In the studies that used this scale, a substantial proportion (at least one-third) of the hypnotic subjects and also of the task motivated subjects indicated that they *saw* the suggested object. The other rating scale permitted the subject to state that he had either *imagined* or *seen* the suggested object. When this scale was used, the great majority of hypnotic subjects and also of task motivated subjects indicated that they had *imagined* it; only a small proportion (about 5-10%) indicated that they had *seen* it.

Another recent experiment (Spanos, Ham & Barber, 1973) clarified some of the problems pertaining to suggested visual hallucinations. In this experiment, the subjects were first individually given suggestions to hallucinate (to see an object that was not actually present) under a control (base-line) condition and then again after they had received either task motivational instructions or a standardized hypnotic induction procedure. During the experiment, the subjects rated the vividness and reality of the suggested object on a scale that permitted them to state that they did not imagine it, they vaguely or vividly imagined it, they saw it, or they saw it and believed part of the time or all of the time that it was "actually out there." The subjects were also interviewed postexperimentally in order to determine what they experienced when they were given the suggestion to hallucinate. In the postexperimental interviews, the subjects were also asked to describe the location, vividness, differential clarity, transparency, and stability of the "hallucinated" object. The results were as follows:

1. When unselected subjects were given the suggestion to hallucinate under a control (base-line) condition (without a hypnotic induction procedure or task motivational instructions), 2% reported that they *saw* the (suggested object. The remaining 98% of the subjects reported that they either vaguely or vividly imagined it or did not imagine it at all.

2. After the subjects were exposed to either a hypnotic induction procedure or task motivational instructions, 8% stated that they *saw* the (suggested) object.

3. In general, the subjects exposed to task motivational instructions were as responsive to the suggestion to hallucinate as those exposed to the hypnotic induction procedure.

4. Some subjects used the terms *imagined* and *saw* interchangeably or were willing to use the term *saw* to refer to their imaginings. For instance, some subjects who used the term *imagine* to describe their experiences during the experiment, later, during the postexperimental interview, used the term *saw* to refer to the same experience.

5. Subjects who had reported during the experiment that they *vividly imagined* the (suggested) object did not differ from those who had

.

reported that they *saw* it in the way they described the location, vividness, differential clarity, transparency, or stability of the "hallucinated" object during the postexperimental interviews.

6. A small number of subjects stated during the experiment that they saw the (suggested) object and, in addition, believed, part of the time, that it was actually there. One percent of the subjects gave these kinds of reports under the control (base-line) condition, 3% under the task motivational condition, and 5% under the hypnotic induction condition. During the postexperimental interviews, these subjects indicated that, when they were given the suggestion to see the object, they concentrated on imagining it and, while doing so, were not concerned with whether or not what they were imagining was "real."

"TRANCE LOGIC"

Orne (1959) presented anecdotal data indicating that "hypnotized" subjects show a unique type of logic, which he labeled *trance logic*. He coined this term to refer to events such as the following: subjects who were judged to be deeply hypnotized stated that (a) they could see a (hallucinated) person sitting in a chair and, at the same time, they could see the chair through the (hallucinated) person and (b) they could see an actual person standing in the room and, at the same time, they could see a hallucination of the same person in another part of the room. Orne's report seemed to support the traditional "hypnotic trance" viewpoint. Since the hypnotic subjects apparently manifested a special type of logic, it appeared reasonable to assume that they were in a "special state."

However, subsequent carefully conducted investigations (Johnson, 1972; Johnson, Maher, & Barber, 1972) showed that nonhypnotic subjects gave these kinds of "illogical" reports to the same extent as subjects who were judged to be "deeply hypnotized." Although "trance logic" was found in some "hypnotic trance" subjects, it was found as often in "unhypnotizable" subjects who were asked to act as if they were hypnotized (to simulate hypnosis) and in control subjects who were simply asked to imagine the (hallucinated) person. In brief, Orne's (1959) interesting anecdotal report, which has received wide publicity, is misleading—the experimental evidence available at present does *not* support the contention that "hypnotized" subjects are characterized by a special type of logic (cf. Blum & Graef, 1971; Hilgard, 1972; Johnson, 1972).[4]

SUMMARY

The wonders that have been associated with hypnotism are said to include (a) the production of perceptual effects such as deafness, blindness, and colorblindness, (b) the elicitation of physiological changes such as the cure of warts, (c) the reinstatement of childhood behaviors and experiences by hypnotic age regression, (d) the production of visual hallucinations, and (e) the elicitation of special cognitive processes such as trance logic. At first glance, these kinds of marvelous effects seem to be more easily explained from the "hypnotic trance" viewpoint than from the cognitive-behavioral viewpoint. A close look at the data, however, does not support an explanation in terms of "hypnotic trance" for several reasons, including the following: Suggestions given to subjects who are said to be in "hypnotic trance" and also suggestions given to control subjects who have not been exposed to a hypnotic induction procedure are at times effective in producing (a) "deafness," "blindness," and "colorblindness," (b) physiological effects such as the cure of warts, (c) behaviors and experiences that ostensibly resemble those found during childhood ("age regression"), (d) vivid visualizing or imagining ("visual hallucination"), and (e) so-called "trance logic."

NOTES

[1] Although suggestions given with or without "hypnotic trance" have been reported to be effective at times in curing warts, much more research is needed to exclude the possibility that the warts would have disappeared spontaneously if no suggestions had been given (Memmesheimer & Eisenlohr, 1931). Another reason why more research is necessary in this area is that several recent, carefully conducted investigations (Clarke, 1965; Stankler, 1967; Tenzel & Taylor, 1969) failed to demonstrate that suggestions given with or without "hypnotic trance" have an effect on warts.

[2] Other physiological effects that have been associated with hypnotism—for example, the production of "blisters"—are discussed in detail elsewhere (Barber, 1970).

[3] A recent study by Parrish, Lundy, and Leibowitz (1969) appeared to indicate that "hypnotic age regression" produces an amazing reinstatement of perceptual responses that are found during childhood. In this study, adult subjects who were "hypnotically regressed" to ages 9 and 5 perceived two optical illusions (the Ponzo and Poggendorff illusions) in very much the same way that they are perceived by 9- and 5-year-old children. Since adults perceive these optical illusions quite differently from children, it appeared that "hypnotic age regression" had reinstated a way of perceiving that was present during childhood.

Although the results of the Parrish et al. experiment are very interesting, they are also open to very serious question. Attempts were made to cross-validate the results in four subsequent experiments: two by Ascher, Barber, and Spanos (1972), one by Perry and Chisholm (1973) and one by Porter, Woodward, Bisbee, and Fenker (1972). Each of these four carefully conducted experiments found that under "hypnotic regression" to ages 9 and 5 subjects perceived the Ponzo or Poggendorff illusions in the same way as adults, not at all in the way they are perceived by children of ages 9 and 5.

[4] Orne and his collaborators have also carried out a series of studies that compared the performance of "real" hypnotic subjects with that of simulating subjects who were asked to try to fool the hypnotist by acting as if they were hypnotized (Evans & Orne, 1971; Nace & Orne, 1970; Orne & Evans, 1966, Orne, Sheehan, & Evans, 1968; Sheehan & Orne, 1968). In these studies, the "real" hypnotic subjects differed from the simulators on the aspect of performance that was under investigation; for instance, the "real" hypnotic subjects, but not the simulators, responded to a posthypnotic suggestion when the hypnotist was not present or they did not open their eyes when the hypnotist left the room. Since the "real" hypnotic subjects differed in a critical behavior from the simulators, Orne and his collaborators concluded that the "real" subjects were in a special state ("hypnotic trance"). This conclusion is not justified. None of the studies used a control group or a task motivated group that was *not* asked to simulate. Although the "real" hypnotic subjects performed differently from the simulators, there is reason to believe that they may not have performed differently from a control group or a task motivated group (Barber, 1969b, pp. 27-28; Barber, 1972; Spanos & Chaves, 1970). Each of the aforementioned studies by Orne and his collaborators needs to be redone with the addition of either control subjects or task motivated subjects who are *not* asked to try to fool the hypnotist by acting as if they are hypnotized (Spanos & Barber, 1973).

* * *

Estabrooks extract is from the book HYPNOTISM by G.H. Estabrooks. Copyright 1943 and 1957 by E.P. Dutton & Co., Inc., publishers and used with their permission.

CHAPTER 8

Hypnotism and Surgical Pain

In 1829, prior to the discovery of anesthetic drugs, a French surgeon, Dr. Cloquet, performed a remarkable operation on a 64-year-old woman who suffered from cancer of the right breast. After making an incision from the armpit to the inner side of the breast, he removed both the malignant tumor and also several enlarged glands in the armpit. What makes this operation remarkable is that, during the surgical procedure, the patient, who had not received any drugs, conversed quietly with the physician and showed no signs of experiencing pain. During the surgery, her respiration and pulse rate appeared stable and there were no noticeable changes in her facial expression. The ability of this patient to tolerate the painful procedures was attributed to the fact that she had been mesmerized immediately prior to the operation. Cloquet's case is one of the first reports of painless surgery with mesmerism or, as it was called later, hypnotism (Chertok, 1959; Kroger, 1957).

Cloquet was subjected to severe criticism when he reported his case to the French Academy of Medicine. Lisfranc, an eminent surgeon of that day, declared that Cloquet was either an imposter or a dupe. Larrey, the former Surgeon-in-Chief of the Grande Armee, claimed that Cloquet had been taken in by trickery. In spite of these criticisms, reports of painless surgery under mesmerism or hypnotism began to appear with some regularity and, in fact, still continue to appear.

Although Cloquet's case clearly indicates that at least some individuals can undergo surgery without manifesting signs of pain, it does not prove that mesmerism or "hypnotic trance" is the important factor in producing this effect. For instance, a very similar operation carried out about the same time, which did not involve mesmerism or hypnotism, has been described by Freemont-Smith (1950). The case involved a woman who had a breast removed for cancer. Since the operation was carried out in the early part of the nineteenth century, before drugs had been discovered that could produce anesthesia (absence of sensitivity) or analgesia (absence of sensitivity to pain), the patient underwent the surgery without medications. The operation took place in a large amphitheater before a group of eminent surgeons. Although the patient was not "hypnotized" and did not receive drugs, she tolerated the surgery ". . . without a word, and after being bandaged up, got up, made a curtsy, thanked the surgeon and walked out of the room."

Later in the nineteenth century, there were other cases of ostensibly painless surgery. For instance, some years later, Tuckey (1889) described the following case:

There are few cases of this kind more remarkable than one related by Mr. Woodhouse Braine, the well-known chloroformist. Having to administer ether to an hysterical girl who was about to be operated on for the removal of two sebaceous tumors from the scalp he found that the ether bottle was empty, and that the inhaling bag was free from even the odor of any anesthetic. While a fresh supply was being obtained, he thought to familiarize the patient with the process by putting the inhaling bag over her mouth and nose, and telling her to breathe quietly and deeply. After a few inspirations she cried, "Oh, I feel it; I am going off," and a moment after, her eyes turned up, and she became unconscious. As she was found to be perfectly insensible, and the ether had not yet come, Mr. Braine proposed that the surgeon should proceed with the operation. One tumor was removed without the least disturbing her, and then, in order to test her condition, a bystander said that she was coming to. Upon this she began to show signs of waking, so the bag was once more applied, with the remark, "She'll soon be off again," when she immediately lost sensation and the operation was successfully and painlessly completed [pp. 725-726].

Unfortunately, all of the early reports of painless surgery are quite anecdotal. Although the patients tolerated the surgery, it was not definitely established that they experienced no pain at all. It does appear likely that pain was markedly reduced, but it remains unclear what factors may have been responsible for the pain reduction.

The foregoing considerations lead to two major questions:

1. To what extent can pain be attenuated by suggestions given with or without a hypnotic induction procedure?
2. What factors are responsible for the reduction of pain?

We shall attempt to answer these questions. However, before we proceed, we need to look briefly at the complexity of pain and at methods that are used to measure it.

THE COMPLEXITY OF PAIN

The term *pain* refers to a variety of sensations—for example, pricking, throbbing, burning, and sharp sensations—that are described as unpleasant. Pain as an unpleasant sensation can vary, quantitatively, from very slight to very intense. However, pain as a sensation is usually closely intermingled with anxiety, fear, worry, anger, and other types of emotions. The total experience of pain thus usually involves a complex blending of unpleasant sensations with emotions.

It appears that when a patient becomes very anxious or fearful while he receives pain-producing stimulation, he tends to report that the pain is more intense. On the other hand, when a patient remains relaxed and does not become anxious about the pain-producing stimulation, he tends to report that the pain is less intense (Barber, 1959; Beecher, 1946, 1956).

Furthermore, it appears that some procedures that are said to reduce pain actually reduce anxiety, fear, worry, and other emotions that are usually intermingled with pain. For instance, the pain relief that follows the administration of morphine and other opiates may be closely related to the reduction in anxiety or fear. Although the patient who has received an opiate may still experience pain sensations, the reduction in anxiety, fear, or other emotions apparently leads him to report that pain is reduced (Barber, 1959, 1970; Beecher, 1959; Cattell, 1943; Hill, Kornetsky, Flanary, & Wilker, 1952a, 1952b; Kornetsky, 1954). Moreover, a surgical procedure—prefrontal lobotomy—that is said to relieve intractable pain, also appears to alter the patient's pain experience primarily by reducing anxiety or fear. Lobotomized patients typically report that they feel pain, but it does not bother them anymore.

MEASUREMENT OF PAIN

Since pain as a sensation is closely interblended with and affected by anxiety, fear, and worry or concern, it is a difficult phenomenon to measure. Clinicians and researchers concerned with the effectiveness of hypnotism or suggestions in relieving pain have used at least three indices to assess pain: verbal reports, physiological measures, and overt behavioral signs. Let us briefly examine these indices.

The patient's verbal report is generally the most informative measure concerning pain (Hilgard, 1969b). Patients can be asked to describe not only the magnitude of their pain but also its quality. Verbal reports can be readily obtained and require no special equipment. Although verbal reports are very useful, under certain conditions (such as when there is strong motivation to deny pain) they may be difficult to interpret. A strong motivation to deny pain may be present when the physician and other medical personnel have invested much time and effort in attempts to alleviate the patient's suffering (Mandy, Mandy, Farkas, & Scher, 1952). This possibility should be considered in evaluating suggested analgesia (suggested removal of pain), because verbal reports are typically used to evaluate pain and the patient may be motivated to deny that pain was experienced.

Investigators at times rely on physiological measures as indicants of pain. These physiological measures, which are commonly altered in normal individuals during painful stimulations, include, for example, blood pressure, heart rate, respiration, skin resistance or conductance, and forehead muscle tension. It should be noted, however, that alterations in these physiological measures during pain-producing stimulation are often closely related to anxiety, fear, anger, and other emotions (Barber & Coules, 1959; Doupe, Miller, & Keller, 1939; Hardy, Wolff, & Goodell, 1952; Levine, 1930; Sattler, 1943). Each of these physiological measures can also be altered by nonpainful stimuli and are especially affected by events that produce anxiety, fear, or emotional arousal. Although physiological measures are useful as indicants of pain when they are used in conjunction with the patient's verbal reports, they are insufficient by themselves to draw conclusions about the quality or degree of the patient's pain.

Investigators also commonly infer the presence of pain when the patient shows overt behavioral signs such as flinching, grimacing, moaning, or withdrawal from the stimulus. However, some patients who report pain can voluntarily inhibit these overt behavioral signs. Consequently, when the signs are absent, we cannot conclude with certainty that the patient is not experiencing pain. Also, patients at times flinch or grimace in *anticipation* of a painful stimulus. Consequently, the presence of the behavioral signs does not necessarily indicate that the patient is experiencing pain.

Taken separately, none of the three indices of pain has proven completely satisfactory. A major difficulty, as implied above, is that the indices are not always closely correlated. Since pain is comprised of a complex intermingling of "sensations" with "emotions," it is difficult to measure and evaluate its reduction by hypnotism and suggestions. Despite these difficulties, we believe that we can clarify some of the effects of hypnotism and suggestions on surgical pain. Let us begin our discussion by looking closely at the severity of the pain sensations that are due to surgical incisions.

SENSATIONS OF PAIN DURING SURGERY

When patients undergo major or even minor surgery, it is usually assumed that it would be impossible for them to tolerate the operation if drugs or special techniques were not used to reduce pain. Moreover, it is commonly assumed that, other things being equal, pain increases when the surgeon cuts into deeper and deeper body tissues and organs. Cutting the skin is thought to be less painful than incising the underlying muscles or the internal organs such as the stomach, liver, or kidney. The available evidence indicates that all of the foregoing assumptions are incorrect. Let us examine these assumptions.

Although surgical procedures give rise to anxiety, fear, worry, and other emotions, they usually give rise to fewer and less intense pain sensations than is commonly believed. Although the skin is very sensitive, the muscles, bone, and most of the internal organs of the body are relatively insensitive. More precisely, the skin is sensitive to a knife cut, but the skilled surgeon cuts through the skin smoothly and quickly and the underlying tissues and internal organs are generally insensitive *to incision*. Lewis (1942) has carefully documented the fact that the muscles, bone, internal organs, and most other parts of the body (with the exception of the skin) are insensitive *to cutting* (although they are generally sensitive to other stimuli such as pulling, traction, or stretching). For instance, he noted the following: The subcutaneous tissue gives rise to little pain when it is cut. Slight pain is elicited when muscles are cut. Compact bone can be bored without pain. The articular surfaces of joints are insensitive. The brain is quite insensitive. The lungs and visceral pleura are insensitive to puncture. The surface of the heart is insensitive. Surgeons have often painlessly removed pieces of the esophageal wall for histological examination. The abdominal viscera in man have been known for over a century to be insensitive to a knife cut. Cutting the great omentum is accomplished painlessly. Solid organs such as the spleen, liver, and kidney can be cut without the patient being aware of it. The stomach may be cut without pain. Lower portions of the alimentary canal, including the jejunum, ileum, and colon, are also insensitive to cutting. The uterus and internal portions of the vagina are also insensitive, although the mouth of the urethra is sensitive. In brief, although "pain receptors" may be found widely throughout the body, and although many tissues and organs of the body give rise to sensations of pain when they are stretched or pulled or when pressure is applied, most tissues and organs of the body (with the notable exception of the skin) give rise to little or no pain sensations when they are cut by the surgeon's scalpel.[1]

In the early 1900's, Lennander (1901, 1902, 1904, 1906a, 1906b) and Mitchell (1907) published a series of case reports indicating that major surgical operations could be accomplished painlessly with the use of only local anesthetics to remove sensitivity from the skin. Lennander performed a large number of abdominal operations using only local anesthetics, such as cocaine, to dull the pain of the initial skin incision. In the vast majority of cases, the remainder of the abdominal operation was accomplished painlessly, even though additional pain-relieving drugs were not used. Lennander consistently reported that the internal organs are insensitive to incision.

Mitchell (1907) also reported an extensive series of major operations performed with local anesthetics that were used to produce insensitivity of the skin. These operations included amputation of limbs, removal of thyroid glands, removal of female breast, removal of the appendix, cutting into and draining the gall bladder, suturing a hernia, excising glands in the neck and groin, and cutting the bladder. In addition, Mitchell noted that very extensive dissection of the neck was possible with the use of only local anesthetics.

Mitchell (1907) also confirmed Lennander's findings regarding the insensitivity of the internal organs. For instance, he wrote as follows:

> The skin being thoroughly anesthetized and the incision being made, there is little sensation in the subcutaneous tissues and muscles as long as the blood vessels, large nerve trunks and connective tissue bundles are avoided. . . . The same insensibility to pain in bone has been noted in several cases of amputation, in the removal of osteophytes and wiring of fractures. In every instance after thorough cocainization of the periostium, the actual manipulations of the bone have been unaccompanied by pain. The patients have stated that they could feel and hear the sawing, but it was as if a board were being sawn while resting upon some part of the body [p. 200].

Taken together, these findings indicate that the pain associated with major surgery is not as great as is commonly supposed. Although many tissues and organs of the body give rise to pain when they are stretched, pulled, or when there is a deficiency in their supply of blood, most tissues and organs of the body (with the notable exception of the skin) give rise to little or no pain when they are cut by the surgeon. Of course, anxiety and fear of being cut play a major role in surgery. Nowadays, surgery is usually carried out with a general anesthesia primarily because of the anxiety and fear that is aroused and because it is difficult to carry out an operation when the patient is tense, when his muscles are not relaxed, and when he does not remain perfectly still. However, if the patient can tolerate the pain associated with the initial incision through the skin, and if he can remain relaxed and still, many major surgical procedures can be accomplished with little additional pain. Moreover, it is clear that the amount of pain that accompanies surgery is not related in any simple way to the extent of the surgical intervention—superficial surgery that involves the sensitive skin can be accompanied by much more pain than cutting compact bone, the cerebral cortex, the liver, and many other rather insensitive organs.

The findings summarized above imply that, in evaluating the effectiveness of any procedure in reducing surgical pain, it is important to have a base-line measure of pain. Thus, in order to determine the degree of pain reduction that is produced by hypnotism and suggestions, it is necessary to compare the results with those obtained with a control group. The control group should undergo the same surgery without drugs and without a hypnotic induction procedure or suggestions of analgesia. No study has utilized a control group comprised of the same kinds of patients undergoing the same kind of surgery. Of course, there are serious ethical and professional objections to using these kinds of controls in a surgical situation. Nevertheless, when controls are lacking, it is impossible to draw definitive conclusions about the degree of pain reduction produced by suggestions, hypnotism, or any other procedures that aim to alleviate pain. It simply cannot be assumed that all surgical procedures are painful.

With the above considerations in mind, we can begin to understand the effects of hypnotism and suggestions on surgical pain. We shall now discuss the following three points in turn:

1. Drugs for the relief of pain are usually used together with hypnotism and suggestions; in these cases, it is not clear to what extent hypnotism and suggestions reduce the pain.
2. The effects of hypnotism during surgery are commonly exaggerated.
3. There are data indicating that suggestions for pain relief given alone are as effective as the same suggestions given together with hypnotic induction procedures in producing a tolerance for pain during surgery.

USE OF PAIN-RELIEVING DRUGS TOGETHER WITH HYPNOTISM AND SUGGESTIONS

In most of the recent surgical cases, the effects of hypnotic induction procedures and suggestions for pain relief were confounded with the use of anesthetic or analgesic drugs. Let us look at a few illustrative cases.

The first case, presented by Werbel (1967), involved the removal of a tumor from the neck of a 69-year-old female patient. Although Werbel attributed the apparent painlessness of the operation to hypnotism, he also stated that "several cubic centimeters of procaine" (Novocain) were injected into the area where the skin was cut. Since the area of the skin incision was numbed by the local anesthetic, it appears possible that the operation might have been equally tolerable if hypnotism had not been used.[2]

In another illustrative case (Crasilneck, McCranie, & Jenkins, 1956), a temporal lobectomy was performed on a 14-year-old girl suffering from epilepsy. The patient was exposed to a hypnotic induction procedure and to suggestions of analgesia. The authors stated that "the scalp line of incision was injected with a 2% solution of procaine." The patient complained of pain when the dura mater was separated from the bone and she required additional local anesthesia. At another point in surgery, "as a blood vessel in the hippocampal region was being coagulated, the patient suddenly awoke from the hypnotic trance." Prior to the completion of the surgery, the patient was given 100 mg. of thiopental sodium intravenously. During most of the surgical procedures—when cutting through the bone of the scalp and into brain tissue—the patient appeared comfortable and did not seem to experience pain. Although the hypnotic induction procedure and the suggestions of analgesia were probably helpful in relaxing this patient and in reducing anxiety and fear, it is questionable whether they produced a marked reduction in pain sensitivity. It should be noted that (a) the patient showed pain, as would be normally expected, when the dura mater was separated from the bone and when a blood vessel was coagulated, (b) the scalp, which is sensitive to incision, was dulled by the use of Novocain, and (c) since compact bone and the brain are generally insensitive to incision, the patient naturally experienced little or no pain when these areas were cut. In brief, this case and also other similar cases (Finer, 1966; Schwarcz, 1965; Werbel, 1965) seem very amazing only when one wrongly assumes that insensitive body tissues such as compact bone and brain tissue are sensitive to cutting and when one fails to note that a local anesthetic was used to dull sensitive areas such as the skin.

In other recent studies, the effects of hypnotic induction procedures and suggestions for pain relief were confounded with the use of a wide variety of drugs including sedatives and local anesthetics. For instance, Marmer (1956, 1957, 1959) used hypnotism together with suggestions aimed at reducing pain in a large number of surgical cases, but these factors were always combined with many drugs that produce relaxation or pain relief. A typical operation reported by Marmer (1956) involved cutting the wall of the chest (thoracotomy) and then cutting out a considerable portion of a lung. (The lung is insensitive to incision.) The patient, a 25-year-old female, was exposed to a hypnotic induction procedure the night before surgery and again just before surgery. In addition to the hypnotic induction procedure and the suggestions for relief of pain, a wide variety of drugs were administered that were designed to produce sedation and to anesthetize the skin. The skin was dulled by infiltrating it with Novocain (25 cc. of 1% procaine hydrochloride). A wide variety of other drugs were also used including Nembutal, Benadryl, Demerol, scopolamine, Surital, and succinyl-choline.[3] Although the hypnotic induction procedure and the suggestions for pain relief were probably effective in reducing anxiety and fear, it is not clear whether they had a direct effect on pain. The apparent lack of pain in this case might have been due to the wide variety of drugs that were used.

Before closing this section, let us look briefly at three additional illustrative cases presented by Betcher (1960). The first case involved an operation for the repair of a hernia. The patient, a 56-year-old male, was exposed to a hypnotic induction procedure the night before surgery and also immediately before surgery. However, the surgery itself was performed under spinal anesthesia. The second case involved a 12-year-old boy who underwent surgical correction of bilateral clubfoot. In this case, hypnotism and suggestions for pain reduction were combined with nitrous oxide and ether. In the third case, a 10-year-old girl underwent plastic surgery to remove scars on the neck. The operation was started after the girl had been exposed to a hypnotic induction procedure and to suggestions of anesthesia for the operative area. However, the patient "began to whimper softly at the incision of the scalpel" and, consequently, she was given drugs that produced "total chemical anesthesia."

In brief, hypnotism and suggestions are rarely used *alone* in present-day surgery. With few exceptions, hypnotism and suggestions are combined with pain-relieving drugs. Although the hypnotic induction procedure and the suggestions for pain relief often seem to be effective in reducing anxiety, fear, and tensions, the drugs seem to play an important role in relieving pain.

EXAGGERATION OF THE EFFECTS OF HYPNOTISM

If we look back at the early reports of painless surgery under mesmerism or hypnotism, we find that, although the procedures apparently reduced anxiety and fear, the extent to which they reduced pain as a sensation may have been exaggerated. For example, in a classic report, Esdaile (1850) stated that he had performed over 300 major operations and numerous minor surgical procedures during a six-year period while he was working in India. His report is frequently cited as demonstrating painless surgery utilizing mesmerism or hypnotism. However, a careful reading of Esdaile's cases indicates that, although anxiety, fear, and other emotions were apparently reduced to a marked degree, the surgery may not have been as painless as has been supposed.

Esdaile's procedures were studied by a commission appointed by the Bengal government (Braid, 1847). Esdaile first selected ten patients to be observed by the commission. However, three of the ten had to be excluded because they could not be mesmerized, even after attempts extending up to 11 days. One of the patients had one side of a double hydrocele (a circumscribed collection of fluid) tapped painlessly while in the "mesmeric state"; however, the same patient had the other side tapped painlessly while awake, so no conclusion could be drawn in this case regarding the efficacy of mesmerism in reducing pain. The remaining six patients underwent major surgery, including amputation and the removal of scrotal tumors, and all six denied experiencing pain. However, three of the six were described in the commission's report as showing ". . . . convulsive movements of the upper limbs, writhing of the body, distortion of the features giving the face a hideous expression of suppressed agony." Two of the remaining patients showed physiological signs, including erratic pulse rates, suggesting the presence of pain. On the basis of the commission's report, it certainly seems possible that Esdaile's surgery was not as painless as has been supposed.

Soon after Esdaile completed his work in India, there was a rapid decline of interest in "mesmeric surgery" due to the discovery of the anesthetic properties of ether, nitrous oxide, and chloroform. Its staunchest advocates remained loyal, however, pointing out the dangers associated with gaseous anesthetics and noting with satisfaction that not a single death during surgery could be attributed to mesmerism!

About 50 years later, toward the end of the nineteenth century, there was a revival of interest in mesmerism or hypnotism, as it was called by that time. Bramwell (1903) reported that he could "sometimes induce anesthesia by suggestion and . . . occasionally performed surgical operations during hypnosis." Most of the cases reported by Bramwell involved minor dental or surgical procedures. A more critical evaluation of the use of hypnotism in surgery was made by Moll (1889), who noted that ". . . a complete analgesia is extremely rare in hypnosis, although authors, copying from one another assert that it is common" (p. 105). Moll also gave his own examples; for instance: ". . . . I once hypnotized a patient in order to open a boil painlessly. I did not succeed in inducing analgesia, but the patient was almost unable to move, so that I could perform the little operation without difficulty" (p. 330). Moll went on to note that "The value of hypnotism for inducing analgesia is not very great. . . . The cases in which hypnotism can be used to make an operation painless are very rare; the care with which every such case is registered by the daily press shows this."

Beginning around 1930 and extending up to the present, interest in the reduction of pain by hypnotism or by suggestions has increased markedly. Numerous clinical reports, several books (Coppolino, 1965; Marmer, 1959;

Werbel, 1965), and a symposium concerning "hypnotic analgesia" (Lassner, 1964) have been published. In most of the cases that have been reported, it appears that anxiety, fear, and worry or concern were reduced, but it is questionable whether there was a marked reduction in pain as a sensation. Let us look at a few examples.

Anderson (1957) performed an abdominal exploration on a 71-year-old male. Since the patient's general condition was poor, contraindicating general anesthesia, it was decided to use hypnotism. The patient underwent intensive hypnotic training sessions for two weeks prior to surgery. The training sessions included rehearsal of the operative procedure. It appears likely that this factor—rehearsing every step of the operation—may be sufficient to reduce anxiety and fear during the operation. During the surgery, the patient "partially broke trance" and, consequently, 5 cc of 2% Penthothal was administered. A common duct stone was then removed. The report did not state how the patient "broke trance," but he presumably showed signs of pain. Physiological measures, such as changes in heart rate, blood pressure, or respiration, were not reported. Also, no mention was made of a verbal report from the patient regarding any pain he might have experienced. Thus, it is impossible to conclude from this report to what extent the sensory experience of pain was reduced. Furthermore, if we assume that pain was significantly reduced, we do not know whether to attribute the reduction to familiarity with the operative procedures obtained during the rehearsals, to the hypnotic induction procedure, to suggestions for pain reduction, to the Pentothal administered during surgery, or to some other variables.

Cooper and Powles (1945) reported using hypnotism to produce analgesia in six minor surgical procedures. Two cases involved infections in the tips of a finger, two involved abscesses in the palms, and two involved abscesses in the armpit. One of these cases was regarded as unsuccessful because of apprehension on the part of the patient. One of the six cases was described in detail since it was regarded as a good example of the successful use of hypnotism. The patient was an 18-year-old soldier who required incision of two abscesses in the armpit. The patient was premedicated with 1 1/2 gr. Nembutal. Subsequently, he was told he would go to sleep because of the sleeping capsule. Suggestions for relaxation, fatigue, and sleep were continued for ten minutes. Additional suggestions were given for anesthesia of the armpit, arm, and shoulder. During the incision, ". . . there was considerable grimacing and some movement of the contralateral shoulder. . . ." Physiological measures were not reported and the patient's verbal report about his experience was not given. Although Cooper and Powles presented this as an exceptionally successful case demonstrating "satisfactory anesthesia," it is not clear to what extent pain as a sensation was reduced. Other investigators (e.g., Finer & Nylen, 1961; Schwarcz, 1965;

Taugher, 1958) also implied that pain was obliterated by hypnotism even though the patients' verbal reports were not presented and either overt behavioral indices or physiological measures suggested that the patients may have experienced pain.

EFFECTS OF SUGGESTIONS OF ANALGESIA GIVEN WITHOUT A HYPNOTIC INDUCTION PROCEDURE

In a large number of studies, suggestions aimed at removing pain sensitivity were given together with the hypnotic induction procedure. Apparently, it was assumed that the surgery could not be carried out if the suggestions for pain relief or analgesia had been given alone, without a hypnotic induction procedure. This assumption is questionable. For instance, Esdaile (1850, pp. 214-215) reported that a few of his surgical patients who had received explicit or implicit suggestions for analgesia, but who could *not* be placed in "mesmeric trance," were able to tolerate major surgery in the same way as patients who had been placed in "mesmeric trance." Let us look at representative recent studies that indicate that suggestions for pain relief or analgesia given without a hypnotic induction procedure may be sufficient for some patients to tolerate surgical procedures.

During World War II, Sampimon and Woodruff (1946) were working under primitive conditions in a prisoner of war hospital near Singapore. Since the supply of anesthetic and analgesic drugs was practically depleted, hypnotism was used for surgery. Two patients could not be "hypnotized"; since the minor surgical procedures (incision for exploration of an abscess cavity and extraction of a tooth) had to be performed without drugs, they proceeded to operate after giving "the mere suggestion of anesthesia." To their surprise, they found that both patients were able to undergo the procedures without complaints and without noticeable signs of pain. Sampimon and Woodruff wrote: "As a result of these two cases two other patients were anesthetized by suggestions only, without any attempt to induce true hypnosis, and both had teeth removed painlessly."

Lozanov (1967) presented a more recent case of surgery in which suggestions of anesthesia were given without a hypnotic induction procedure. The patient was a 50-year-old man who required surgical repair of a hernia in the groin. Since he was ". . . convinced of the anaesthetizing power of suggestion," he offered to undergo surgery without drugs and without hypnotism. Before the surgery, he was given preparatory practice that involved breathing exercises. The patient did not appear to experience pain during the initial surgical incision—12 cm. in the right groin—or when the muscle tissue was cut. Lozanov reported that "Pain appeared when the process of separation reached the testis. It became necessary to suspend the operation for one minute during which time the patient was subject to additional suggestions." Pain also appeared later "during the broaching of ligamentum inguinale and the periostium of tuberculum pubicum." At that point, 12 cc. of 0.5% Novocain was injected and the remainder of the operation was performed apparently without pain. Lozanov noted that pain was apparently present during two minutes of the 50-minute operation.

In brief, there is evidence to indicate that suggestions for pain relief given *without* "hypnosis" may at times be as effective as suggestions for pain relief given *with* "hypnosis" in producing a tolerance for pain during surgery.

RECAPITULATION

It appears that with the exception of the skin, which is very sensitive, most tissues and organs of the body are rather insensitive to *surgical incisions*. Consequently, if a person is able to tolerate the pain that is associated with the initial skin incision, he might then be able to undergo the rest of the surgery into tissues and organs that lie below the skin without experiencing much severe pain.

With the above facts in mind, reports of surgery performed with the use of hypnotism and suggestions are not as amazing as they first appear. Furthermore, they become even less amazing when we realize that (a) the effectiveness of hypnotism is reducing surgical pain has been exaggerated, (b) in the great majority of cases, *analgesic or anesthetic drugs* were used along with the hypnotism and the suggestions, and (c) although some patients were able to tolerate the surgery, they very commonly showed behavioral or physiological signs of pain, especially when those tissues were cut—for example, the skin or the area near the testis—which are normally quite sensitive.

The studies summarized in this chapter, together with other studies (e.g., Finer, 1966; Hoffman, 1959; Kroger, 1957; Kroger & DeLee, 1957; Mason, 1955; Reis, 1966; Wallace & Coppolino, 1960), indicate that, with at least a small proportion of patients, suggestions aimed at reducing pain given with or without hypnotic induction procedures are sufficient for the patients to tolerate the surgery, to minimize anxiety, fear, and other emotions, and probably to reduce (but not necessarily obliterate) the sensory experience of pain. This conclusion is in line with the results of recent experimental studies pertaining to the reduction of pain, to which we now turn.

EXPERIMENTAL STUDIES ON PAIN REDUCTION

Over the last 40 years, a number of investigators have attempted to clarify the phenomenon of suggested analgesia by bringing it into the laboratory. In these experiments, a wide range of procedures have been used to produce pain, including pressure from a sharp point, electric shock, radiant heat, immersion of a limb in ice cold water, occlusion of the blood supply to a limb, and application of a heavy weight to the bony part of a finger (cf. Barber, 1970). Obviously, the pain produced by these stimuli may differ in quality and may give rise to less anxiety and fear than the pain of surgery. However, it appears possible that some kinds of pain produced in the laboratory—for instance, the pain produced by occlusion of the blood supply to a limb or by application of a heavy weight to the bony part of a finger—may be as intense as the pain that is found during some surgical procedures.

Although the pain produced in the laboratory generally gives rise to less anxiety and fear than the pain produced by the surgeon's scalpel, it is nevertheless possible to draw some conclusions from the laboratory studies that are relevant to understanding how some patients are able to tolerate surgery without receiving drugs. Let us briefly state these generalizations before going on to examine the supporting data.

1. Implicit or explicit suggestions for pain relief or analgesia are effective in reducing reported pain regardless of whether or not a hypnotic induction procedure has been administered.
2. Reported pain is reduced when the subjects are distracted during the pain-producing stimulation.
3. Subjects report less pain when they are asked to imagine situations— e.g., to imagine a limb as a piece of rubber—which, if they actually occurred, would be incompatible with the experience of pain.
4. Subjects who are not anxious report less pain than those who are anxious and fearful.

Let us examine some of the data that support these generalizations.

Suggestions for Anesthesia or for Relief of Pain

Hilgard and his associates (Hilgard, 1967; Hilgard, Cooper, Lenox, Morgan, & Voevodsky, 1967; Morgan, Lezard, Prytulak, & Hilgard, 1970) confirmed earlier observations indicating that hypnotic subjects who have received suggestions of anesthesia report less pain than control subjects who have not received suggestions of anesthesia. However, several recent studies (Barber, 1969a; Evans & Paul, 1970; Spanos, Barber, & Lang, 1969), which will be discussed next, showed that, if nonhypnotic subjects are also exposed to suggestions of anesthesia, they show as much reduction in pain as hypnotic subjects who are exposed to the same suggestions of anesthesia.

Barber (1969a) gave identical suggestions of anesthesia ("Your hand is numb and insensitive . . .") to two groups of subjects—a group that had been exposed to a standardized hypnotic induction procedure and a group that had not been exposed to an induction. The pain stimulus was a heavy weight applied to the bony part of a finger for one minute. As compared to a no-suggestions condition (control group), the suggestions of anesthesia were effective in reducing reported pain in both the hypnotic and the nonhypnotic subjects. Moreover, the magnitude of the pain reduction was about the same in both the hypnotic and the nonhypnotic groups.

Spanos, Barber, and Lang (1969) confirmed the above results. These investigators also gave suggestions of anesthesia ("Your hand is numb and insensitive . . .") to subjects who had, and also to those who had not, been exposed to a standardized hypnotic induction procedure. The pain stimulus was again a heavy weight applied to the bony part of a finger. Again, as compared to control groups that did not receive any suggestions, the suggestions of anesthesia were effective in producing an equal reduction in reported pain in the hypnotic subjects and the nonhypnotic subjects. Most of the hypnotic and nonhypnotic subjects who received the suggestions of anesthesia showed a small reduction in reported pain and about one-fourth of these subjects showed a moderate reduction (3 or more points on a 10-point scale).

Evans and Paul (1970) cross-validated the above results in an experiment in which pain was produced by immersion of the hand in ice water at 0 to 2°C. Suggestions of anesthesia ("Your hand has no feeling at all . . .") were given to subjects who had been exposed to a hypnotic induction procedure and also to subjects who had not been exposed to an induction. Other subjects, assigned to control groups, were not given suggestions of anesthesia. The hypnotic and nonhypnotic subjects who received suggestions of anesthesia reported less pain than the control groups. Also, the hypnotic induction procedure was irrelevant in reducing pain; the two groups of subjects who received suggestions of anesthesia—hypnotic subjects and nonhypnotic subjects—reported the same degree of pain reduction.

Clinical studies also indicate that implicit suggestions for pain relief, given without hypnotic induction procedures, are effective in reducing pain in a substantial proportion of patients. For instance, pain was reduced when placebos were given with the implication that pain relief should be expected. Beecher

(1955) and his associates (Lasagna, Mosteller, von Felsinger, & Beecher, 1954) found that satisfactory relief of pain, defined as "50 percent or more relief of pain at 45 and 90 minutes after administration of the agent," could be achieved with placebos in 35% of their postsurgical patients. These findings were confirmed in similar studies by Houde and Wallenstein (1953) and Keats (1956). Furthermore, Laszlo and Spencer (1953) found that "over 50% of patients who had received analgesics for a long period of time could be adequately controlled by placebo medication."

The data summarized above, and other data reviewed elsewhere (Barber, 1959, 1963, 1970), support the notion that explicit and implicit suggestions for pain relief tend to reduce anxiety, fear, and also the degree of reported pain in experimental subjects and in clinical patients.

The Role of Distraction

When attempts are made to produce "hypnotic analgesia," the patients are at times given instructions designed to focus their attention on something other than the painful stimulus. The available data suggest that a wide variety of distractions are effective in reducing pain (Barber, 1969a; Barber & Cooper, 1972; Barber & Hahn, 1962; Gammon & Starr, 1941; Gammon, Starr, & Bronk, 1936; Kanfer & Goldfoot, 1966; Notermans, 1966, 1967).

In one of these experiments (Barber, 1969a), student nurses were exposed to pain-producing stimulation (a heavy weight applied to a finger) while they listened to a tape recording that presented the interesting erotic escapades of an unnamed Hollywood actor. They were asked to guess the identity of the actor and to remember as many of the details of his escapades as possible. Immediately prior to the pain stimulation, some of the subjects had been exposed to a standardized hypnotic induction procedure and others had not. The distraction of listening to the interesting tape recording produced a significant reduction in reported pain. It is particularly interesting to note that the magnitude of the pain reduction was the same in both the hypnotic and nonhypnotic subjects. Similarly, in another recent study (Barber & Cooper, 1972), two distractions—listening to an interesting tape recorded story and adding numbers aloud—were both effective in reducing the degree of reported pain. An earlier study (Kanfer & Goldfoot, 1966) also showed that pain was reduced by three distractors (verbalizing the sensations aloud, self-pacing with a clock, and observing a series of slides).

Other kinds of distractions also appear to be effective in reducing the degree of reported pain. For instance, Notermans (1966) found that pain was apparently reduced when the subjects were engaged in the distracting task of inflating a manometer cuff and also when they were distracted by another noxious stimulus applied to another part of the body.

In brief, the available studies suggest that distraction can attenuate pain. Moreover, the distraction can either take the form of external stimulation or instructing the subjects to direct their attention to something besides the pain-producing stimulus.

Cognitive Strategies

It also appears that certain kinds of "cognitive strategies" are useful in reducing pain. These strategies involve imagining situations which, if real, would result in the reduction or elimination of pain. For example, when a pain-producing stimulus is applied to a finger, the subject might try to think of pleasant events or might try to think and imagine that the finger is numb and insensitive (Spanos, Barber, & Lang, 1969).

Barber and Hahn (1962) showed that one kind of cognitive strategy—thinking of previously-experienced pleasant events—significantly reduced reported pain caused by the immersion of a hand in ice cold water (at $2°C.$). Two physiological correlates of pain—irregular pattern of respiration and forehead muscle tension—were also diminished. The nonhypnotic subjects who thought of pleasant events during the painful stimulation showed the same degree of reduction in pain experience as "good" hypnotic subjects who had been exposed to a hypnotic induction procedure and to suggestions of anesthesia.

Chaves and Barber (in press) compared the degree of pain reduction that could be achieved by using two different cognitive strategies—imagining that a finger is insensitive and imagining pleasant events. In addition, other subjects were led to expect a reduction in pain but were not provided with any cognitive strategies. The subjects who were simply led to expect a reduction in pain, in fact, did report less pain than uninstructed control subjects. However, even greater pain reductions were shown by subjects who were asked to use the cognitive strategies for reducing pain—that is, who were instructed to imagine that the finger was insensitive or to imagine pleasant events.

In summary, a number of procedures are effective in reducing experimentally-produced pain including direct suggestions of anesthesia, distraction, leading subjects to expect a reduction in pain, as well as providing subjects with cognitive strategies for pain reduction.

Reduction of Anxiety and Fear

As stated at the beginning of this chapter, in the surgical situation and to a lesser degree in the laboratory, the experience of pain is usually closely intermingled with fear, anxiety, worry, and other emotions. There is evidence indicating that relief of postoperative pain due to the administration of morphine as well as placebos may be more closely related to the alleviation of fear or anxiety rather than to a marked alteration in the pain sensations (Barber, 1959;

Beecher, 1959; Cattell, 1943). Even neurosurgical procedures designed to alleviate intractable pain, such as prefrontal lobotomy, seem to reduce anxiety and
fear without markedly altering the pain sensations.

The reduction in anxiety and fear seems to dramatically reduce the overall
pain experience. Many investigators appear to agree with Ostenasek's (1948)
conclusion that ". . . . when the fear of pain is abolished, the perception of pain
is not intolerable."

Implications

In brief, it appears that a wide variety of procedures are capable of reducing
pain. The variables mentioned above may also play an important role in producing the apparent reduction in pain that has been associated with hypnotism. To
illustrate this contention, let us look briefly at the effects of distraction. The
hypothesis that distraction plays an important role in reducing pain in "hypnotized" subjects was proffered many years ago by Liebeault (1885). He contended that, when suggestions are effective in reducing pain in hypnotic subjects,
the mediating process involves a focusing of attention on thoughts or ideas other
than those concerning pain. More recently, a similar conclusion was reached by
August (1961) after a large-scale investigation of 1000 patients during childbirth.
August concluded that hypnotic induction procedures and suggestions are effective in reducing pain during childbirth to the extent that they "direct attention
away from pain responses to pleasant ideas" (p. 62).

Of course, distraction is not the only factor and may not be the most
important factor in reducing pain in hypnotic situations. Hypnotic subjects are
explicitly or implicitly led to believe that they are undergoing a procedure that
will attenuate pain and attempts are made to reduce anxiety and fear. Furthermore, they are given various types of suggestions and instructions and some of
these suggestions may give rise to "cognitive strategies" that are effective in
attenuating pain. Also, a close interpersonal relationship may exist between the
patient and the hypnotist. This relationship could affect the kinds of pain
reports that are obtained from the patients (Barber, 1970, pp. 239-240; Egbert,
Battit, Turndorf, & Beecher, 1963; Egbert, Battit, Welch, & Bartlett, 1964).[4]

Suggestions for Further Research

Although we have pointed to a number of variables that appear to play an
important role in pain, a number of questions remain unanswered. One of the
most striking questions pertains to individual differences. Some individuals seem
to be able to adopt a detached attitude toward pain, treating it in the same way
as other sensations and not being especially bothered by it. On the other hand,
other individuals are hyperreactive to pain and are extremely disturbed by

relatively minor pain-producing stimulation. A major research problem in this area is to identify the variables that produce these differences. If these variables could be specified, we might successfully train a large proportion of individuals to tolerate painful stimuli (see Chapter 10).

Some success has already been achieved. Experimental data indicate that pain can be reduced by minimizing subjects' anxiety, by leading subjects to expect that they have the ability to control pain, by asking subjects to imagine situations that are incompatible with the experience of pain, by distracting the subjects, and by administering suggestions for pain reduction. Clearly, much additional work is needed to utilize these variables effectively in controlling pain. For example, what kinds of procedures are most effective in producing distraction? How can the effective variables be implemented in teaching tolerance of pain? Preliminary efforts aimed at teaching individuals to control pain are discussed in Chapter 10.

SUMMARY

One of the most striking phenomena associated with hypnotism is its use in controlling the pain of surgery. This chapter has attempted to place this dramatic phenomenon in perspective by emphasizing that most tissues and organs of the body, with the notable exception of the skin, are rather insensitive to the surgeon's scalpel. Many individuals can tolerate the pain of surgery if local anesthetics such as Novocain are used to dull the skin for the initial incision. In addition, experimental and clinical data indicate that pain is reduced when the patients have low levels of anxiety and fear, when they have positive attitudes, motivations, and expectancies about the situation, when they are distracted, when they are given suggestions for analgesia or for pain reduction, and when they utilize a variety of "cognitive strategies" for pain reduction, such as thinking and imagining that the stimulated body part is a piece of rubber or is numb and insensitive. When some or many of these factors are present—in hypnotic situations, in nonhypnotic situations such as those described by Lozanov (1967) and others (Freemont-Smith, 1950; Sampimon & Woodruff, 1946; Tuckey, 1889, pp. 725-726), and also in acupuncture situations (see Appendix B)—some individuals are able to tolerate surgical pain.[5]

NOTES

[1] Although *most* tissues and organs of the human body are rather insensitive when they are cut, the surgeon's incision does produce pain when it cuts the skin and other external tissues such as the conjunctiva, the mucous membranes of the mouth and nasopharynx, the upper surface of the larynx, and the stratified mucous membranes of the genitalia. Also, it appears that a small number of deeper tissues, such as the deep fascia, the peritoneum, the periostium, the tendons, and the rectum, hurt when they are cut (Lewis, 1942).

[2] Other present-day investigators also use hypnotism together with local anesthetics during surgery. For instance, Van Dyke (1965) presented a case of a 9-year-old boy who was operated on for a bony cyst in the jaw which was delaying the descent of a permanent canine tooth. Prior to the surgery, the boy was given two training sessions in hypnosis. Immediately before the operation, he was exposed to a hypnotic induction procedure and to suggestions aimed at relieving pain. Although no preoperative medication was used, an unspecified amount of Novocain was administered immediately before surgery, making it difficult to determine to what extent the relief of pain was due to the hypnotic induction procedure, to the suggestions for pain relief, or to the use of Novocain. Similarly, Van Dyke presented another case involving surgical incision of the female vulvar orifice (episiotomy) in which the effects of hypnotism and suggestions in alleviating pain were confounded with the effects of 5 cc. of Novocain.

[3] In addition to the use of Novocain, the following drugs were administered to the patient: 0.10 gm. pentobarbital (Nembutal), 50 mg. diphenhydramine hydrochloride (Benadryl), 100 mg. meperidine hydrochloride (Demerol), 0.40 mg. scopolamine, and 50 mg. thiamylal sodium (Surital). Also, during dissection of the lung, 100 mg. of a 0.1% solution of succinylcholine was administered.

[4] Our analysis suggests that there are a host of variables that are effective in reducing pain. If these variables have broad relevance, we should also be able to see their effects in faith healing, in exorcism, in acupuncture, and in other situations in which pain is ostensibly reduced without the use of drugs. In Appendix B, we look at one of these techniques—the use of acupuncture in surgery—to see whether the variables that we have outlined in this chapter are helpful in understanding this technique for alleviating surgical pain.

[5] In this chapter, we have focused on *surgical pain*. The effects of hypnotism and suggestions on other kinds of pain—e.g., labor pain, postsurgical pain, and pain associated with cancer—are discussed by Barber (1970, Chap. 5).

* * *

Mitchell extract is from Mitchell, J.F. Local anesthesia in general surgery. *Journal of the American Medical Association*, 1907, 48, 198-201.

Moll extract is from Moll, Albert. *The Study of Hypnosis*. New York: Julian Press, 1958.

CHAPTER 9

Stage Hypnotism

Most laymen and many professional psychologists seem to believe that in demonstrations of stage hypnotism the subjects behave in a very special way because they are in a special state ("hypnotic trance"). In fact, much of the lore about "hypnotic trance" seems to derive from the performances that are observed in stage hypnotism. However, appearances are at times misleading and especially so in the case of stage demonstrations. Let us look closely at what actually occurs in stage hypnotism.

The most important principle of stage hypnotism is that the stage performer very carefully picks his subjects (Meeker & Barber, 1971).[1] He uses only selected individuals who are ready to think and imagine with suggestions and to comply with requests and commands. The procedure used by the stage performer to select responsive subjects is clear-cut. He gives several test suggestions to individuals who volunteer to come up to the stage. Although the test suggestions can vary widely, they typically include limb rigidity or hand clasp. For instance, the stage hypnotist asks his volunteers to clasp their hands together tightly and then suggests repeatedly and emphatically that the hands are rigid, solid, stuck together, and cannot be taken apart. He selects only those volunteers who respond to the test suggestion—that is, who struggle to take their hands apart but do not do so until he states, "Now you can relax the hands and you can unclasp them."

Since many of the volunteers pass the first test, the stage hypnotist usually has too many subjects at this point. Consequently, he goes on to give a second test suggestion and, if necessary, a third. The stage performer might suggest that the subject cannot open his mouth, cannot move a leg, or that his eyes are closing and he cannot open them. Volunteers who fail one or more of the tests are sent back to the audience and only those remain on the stage who have passed all of the test suggestions. *The Encyclopedia of Stage Hypnotism* (McGill, 1947, pp. 181-182 and p. 252) places heavy emphasis on this aspect, stating that the stage hypnotist should diplomatically get rid of uncooperative subjects by whispering to them to leave the stage quietly. *The Encyclopedia* also emphasizes that the removal of "poor" subjects is the first thing the stage hypnotist must learn in order to carry out a successful show.

In brief, the stage performer carefully selects subjects who are ready to respond to his suggestions and to accept his requests and commands. He can select these subjects by administering repeated suggestions of relaxation, drowsiness, sleep, and hypnosis. However, the relaxation-sleep-hypnosis suggestions are typically used in the same way as other test suggestions. That is, if the subject does not pass the test suggestion—if he does not appear relaxed and sleepy—he is not used in the demonstration but is sent back to the audience. Although the stage hypnotist does not need to give suggestions of relaxation and deep sleep, he usually does so for at least three reasons: (a) it is expected by the subjects, (b) it impresses the audience, and (c) it formally defines the situation as hypnosis with the strong implication that the situation is both unusual and important.

However, sophisticated stage hypnotists are aware that repeated relaxation-sleep-hypnosis suggestions are not necessary to elicit a high level of suggestibility from volunteer subjects. Lonk (1947) emphasized that "The subject need not be in any stage of sleep. Sleep is not always necessary for the production of the suggestible stage" (p. 34). Tracy (1952) appropriately pointed out that "A good hypnotic subject will respond to many suggestions just as quickly in the waking state. . . . Your confidence and your commanding tone of voice are all that is necessary" (p. 152). Similarly, Arons (1961) has discussed the use of the "waking state" in stage hypnotism and has emphasized that "This phase of the demonstration illustrates forcibly that the hypnotic 'trance' is not needed to perform a hypnotic demonstration" (p. 10). Along similar lines, *The Encyclopedia of Stage Hypnotism* noted how direct suggestions given in the "waking state" can be effective in producing an inability to separate the hands, an inability to close one's mouth, a forgetting of one's name, getting "drunk" on a glass of water, and "hallucinating" a mouse (McGill, 1947, p. 28)

The stage performer can give direct requests or commands to his selected subjects—for example, "Sing like Frank Sinatra" or "You are Frank Sinatra" —and the subjects almost certainly will comply. Some of the reasons for the subjects' compliance include the following: (a) The subjects have been carefully selected for readiness to respond to suggestions, requests, or commands. Stated differently, individuals who have negative attitudes, motivations, and expectancies toward the stage situation and who are unwilling to think and imagine with the themes of the suggestions either do not volunteer for the stage performance or are excluded from the performance during the process of subject selection. (b) The stage performer has been advertised as a highly effective hypnotist and has high prestige and strong expectations working for him. (c) The stage performer will carefully observe his selected subjects and ask the one who appears to be the most highly motivated and the most extroverted to sing like Frank Sinatra. (d) Since the subject is facing an eager and expectant audience and is surrounded by other eager subjects, he would have to be highly negativistic to surmount the pressure and to say to the stage performer: "I will not sing" or "I am not Frank Sinatra." Nelson (1965, p. 30) has emphasized that a subject finds it difficult to refuse a request or command because, if he refused, he would stand out among the other subjects as a "hold out." Also, Nelson (1965, p. 30) noted that the subject "gets into the act," "falls into the fun idea," acts the part of a hypnotized subject, realizes that he has " a perfect shield to hide behind"— namely, "hypnosis"—if he engages in odd or silly behavior, is reinforced by the reactions and applause of the audience, and begins competing with the other subjects for the best performance.

It should be noted that the stage hypnotist utilizes a series of social-psychological variables that are present in the stage situation. *The Encyclopedia of Stage Hypnotism* describes some of these variables as follows: the subject is clearly in a submissive role while the stage hypnotist has the role of the leader or stage director; the attention and expectancy of the audience are centered upon the subject; the subject feels tense and expectant while he is on the stage; and there is a helpful stage "atmosphere" which derives from the lights, music, curtains, and other stage props (McGill, 1947, p. 257). *The Encyclopedia* also points out that some of the subjects tend to simulate, but the simulation is not "voluntary deception"; on the contrary, it derives from a strong desire to cooperate and to "help out the show" (McGill, 1947, p. 257).

It should be emphasized that the audience does not always hear everything that the stage performer says to his subjects. Since the audience is some distance away, the performer can prevent the audience from hearing such statements as "Sing like Frank Sinatra" by simply whispering his statement or by turning away his microphone. However, the audience will be allowed to hear the next statement, which might be: "You are Frank Sinatra!" In other words, the stage performer can mislead the audience into believing that the subject is deluded (thinks he is Frank Sinatra) when actually the subject is responding to a direct request to imitate the singer.

The Encyclopedia of Stage Hypnotism repeatedly emphasizes that the proficient performer allows the audience to hear only some of the interaction that transpires on the stage. For instance, *The Encyclopedia* points out that, when the subject is receiving suggestions for body sway, the stage performer should whisper, "Let yourself go and don't resist. Let yourself come right back towards me . . ." (McGill, 1947, p. 150). *The Encyclopedia* also emphasizes that these intimate whispers to the subject are very important because the subject receives "full benefit of your confidence," which makes him feel obligated to carry out the requests, suggestions, and commands (McGill, 1947, p. 150).

Let us now turn to the unusual case when the stage hypnotist asks the selected subject to carry out an act—e.g., "Dance with an invisible partner"—and the subject refuses to comply. The proficient stage performer will not be especially bothered by such a refusal. Typically, he will simply ask the subject to leave the stage and will work with a more compliant subject. The stage performer can also use another tactic at this point. He can tell the subject, "Please sit down and then please close your eyes," and he can prevent the audience from hearing this polite request. It is very likely that the subject will comply with the polite request and, when he is sitting down and closing his eyes, the stage performer can make hand motions over him and intone aloud so that the audience hears, "You are going into a deep hypnotic trance." Thus, the proficient performer can turn the situation to his advantage—he can lead the audience to believe that he placed the subject in a "trance" in a very quick and amazing way.

Schneck (1958) has shown how some stage hypnotists use another technique—"the failure to challenge technique"—to lead the audience to believe that unusual events are occurring. When using this technique, the stage performer may suggest to the subject that he cannot take his clasped hands apart or he cannot bend his outstretched arm, but he does *not* challenge the subject to try to unclasp his hands or to try to bend his arm. Instead, he simply tells the subject after a few seconds that he can now unclasp his hands or can bend his arm. Members of the audience, however, assume that the suggestions were effective even though they were not tested. Schneck (1958) appropriately pointed out, with respect to the suggestion that the arm cannot be bent, that:

> The point to be noted is the play on the suggestibility of the audience rather than the examination of the subject response. The implication was to the effect that when the subject retained, even for a few seconds, the arm in an outstretched position, it followed that he would in fact be unable to bend it. This was clearly a non-sequitur. No verbal or other response at this point was requested of the subject [p. 175].

The stage hypnotist can also make his show exciting and impressive by having his subjects demonstrate several "amazing feats" that are actually rather easy to perform. For instance, he can suspend one of his subjects between two chairs, one chair beneath the subject's head and neck and the other beneath the ankles. As the subject remains suspended between the two chairs, the stage performer can ask the orchestra to play a crescendo or he can try to impress the audience by stating that the subject is able to perform the human plank feat because he is in "a cataleptic third stage of somnambulistic trance." Of course, trained stage hypnotists know (but very few if any members of the audience know) that practically anyone at any time can rather easily remain suspended between two chairs (one chair beneath the head and neck and the other beneath the ankles). Even though the body is suspended, it is not especially difficult, it does not require any special effort, and practically no one falls. After about two or three minutes, the neck muscles begin to tire and most normal individuals and also "hypnotized" individuals wish to discontinue the "human plank feat" (Barber, 1969b; Collins, 1961).

After the audience is impressed by the "feat" described above, the stage hypnotist can demonstrate another "human plank feat" that appears even more amazing. In this case, he places a male subject between two chairs, one chair beneath the subject's *head and shoulders* and the other beneath the *calves of his legs*. The male subject is told to keep his body rigid. The stage performer then asks the most attractive girl he has available to stand on the chest of the suspended subject. He then takes the girl by the hand and helps her to stand upon the subject's chest. The audience is impressed, especially when the stage performer tells the audience that the reason that the subject is able to support the weight of the girl on his body is because he is in a "profound, somnambulistic, hypnotic trance." Of course, the well-trained stage hypnotist knows (but very few individuals in his audience know) that, when a normal man is suspended between two chairs, he can support at least 300 pounds on his chest without experiencing much discomfort. If the girl "misses" the subject's chest and stands on his abdomen, the performance will still go on except, in this case, the performer will take the girl off more quickly because the subject may be quite uncomfortable when the weight is on his abdomen (and the weight may possibly damage his internal organs). Of course, if the girl steps on the subject's chest as instructed, the stage performer can keep her there for a longer period of time.

The stage hypnotist can make his demonstration even more dramatic by placing a felt pad and then a large stone on the chest of the suspended subject and then breaking the stone by striking a blow with a large, impressive sledgehammer. Although this stunt appears very dramatic to the audience, McGill (1947, p. 219) notes that, since the rock is made of sandstone, it breaks easily. The subject experiences only a slight jar because the force of the blow is absorbed by the felt pad over the subject's chest and by the inertia in the rock itself (McGill, 1947, p. 219).

Other stage demonstrations—for instance, tests of "anesthesia"—are also not what they superficially appear to be. After the stage hypnotist has asked one of his selected subjects to place his hand straight out horizontally, he may state repeatedly that the hand is dull, numb, and insensitive. The stage hypnotist need not care whether the subject experiences the suggested insensitivity because what he is about to demonstrate is not dependent on the subject's experiencing the suggested effect. The stage performer takes a match or a cigarette lighter and places the flame close to or upon the subject's outstretched palm and then moves the flame slowly across the palm. Although this demonstration impresses the audience, the experience stage performer knows that when a flame is held close to the subject's palm or is placed directly upon the palm, no burning results *as long as the flame is moved along slowly*. Although the subject experiences heat, it is not too uncomfortable. Any normal individual can tolerate the heat, and no burning results (Meeker & Barber, 1971).

Next, the stage performer may take a sterilized pin and quickly push it through the loose skin in the middle of the subject's arm. Stage hypnotists learn to do this quickly, without informing the subject, and usually when the subject's eyes are closed (McGill, 1947). They know that, although the finger tips and most parts of the hand are quite sensitive to a pinprick, the fleshy part of the arm is rather insensitive. At best, the subject will feel a tiny prick on the arm, which he can easily tolerate; if the subject is distracted, he may not notice it at all. To make this demonstration dramatic, the stage performer uses a fine needle with a large head.

As implied above, in stage hypnotism it is not especially important whether the subjects experience those things that are suggested. Also, as Nelson (1965, pp. 29-31) bluntly noted, the proficient stage hypnotist does not care whether his subjects are "hypnotized." If he excludes uncooperative subjects and carefully selects only cooperative subjects, he can carry out an entertaining show without caring whether any of the subjects are "hypnotized" or are experiencing those things that are suggested.

SUMMARY

Most laymen, and also many professional psychologists, seem to believe that in demonstrations of stage hypnotism the subjects behave in a very special way because they are in a very special state ("hypnotic trance"). This notion is misleading. The basic principle of stage hypnotism is that the performer carefully selects subjects who are ready to respond to his suggestions and to carry out his requests and commands. Furthermore, since the situation is emphatically defined as hypnotism, it is clear to all of the selected subjects that obedience to suggestions, requests, and commands is desired and expected. In addition, unique characteristics of the stage situation—the expectancy centered on each subject by the audience together with the "fun" atmosphere—are helpful in eliciting obedience. Although these features of the stage situation are sufficient to elicit most of the ostensibly amazing behaviors, stage hypnotists also *at times* use the following to enhance the dramatic nature of their show: the technique of "private whispers," the "failure to challenge technique," and one or more "feats" (such as the human-plank feat and the pin through the flesh test) that seem "amazing" but are actually easy to perform.

NOTES

[1] We are deeply indebted to William Meeker for invaluable assistance in formulating the principles of stage hypnotism.

PART E

Implications and Prospects

CHAPTER 10

Implications for
Human Capabilities and Potentialities

We have contrasted the traditional approach to hypnotism with an alternative approach that we have called the cognitive-behavioral viewpoint. We have examined some of the differences between these two approaches in terms of the nature of so-called hypnotic behaviors, the conditions that are effective in eliciting the behaviors, and the mediating variables involved in their execution. Our discussion has suggested that a major difficulty with the traditional "hypnotic trance" approach is that it consistently underestimates the cognitive-behavioral capabilities open to normal individuals. In the present chapter, we shall explore more fully what these capabilities are and how they might be enhanced.

We shall first present data indicating that individuals who cannot be said to be in a "hypnotic trance" have a wide range of capabilities that are commonly regarded as outside of the normal repertoire. The kind of capabilities we have in mind include the ability (a) to control pain, (b) to feel as if earlier events have been forgotten (amnesia), (c) to control nocturnal dreaming, (d) to control the temperature of the skin, (e) to increase visual acuity, and (f) to control allergic responses. In the first part of this chapter, we shall examine these capabilities. In the second part, we shall outline some specific methods that might be used to train individuals to utilize their capabilities and potentialities.

CONTROL OF PAIN

As stated in Chapter 8, some hypnotic subjects and also some control subjects who have been given suggestions for anesthesia or analgesia do not seem anxious or distressed when exposed to stimuli that are normally painful. In our own experiments in this area (Barber, 1969a; Barber & Hahn, 1962; Spanos, Barber, & Lang, 1969), nursing students or college students were first exposed to stimulation that they experienced as painful; the stimuli involved either the application of a heavy weight on a finger (Forgione & Barber, 1971) or the immersion of a hand in ice water. The subjects were then tested for response to the same pain-producing stimulation a second time. Before receiving the second test, half of the subjects were exposed to a standardized hypnotic induction procedure and the other half, used as controls, were not exposed to a hypnotic induction. Some of the hypnotic subjects and also some of the control subjects, chosen at random, then received the second pain test in exactly the same way as the first (no-suggestion groups). The other hypnotic and control subjects were given the second pain test after receiving either (a) suggestions to think of other things or of pleasant things during the stimulation or (b) suggestions to imagine that the stimulated area was numb and insensitive. The hypnotic subjects and also the control subjects who had received one of the latter two types of suggestions generally showed a reduction in reported pain as compared to the no-suggestion groups. That is, most of the hypnotic and control subjects who received one of the two types of suggestions reported a moderate reduction in pain, and a small proportion reported no pain at all. In contrast, the subjects who did not receive suggestions reported that the stimulation was experienced as painful.

Why did some of the hypnotic and control subjects succeed in reducing their experience of pain? After conducting the experiments summarized above and also other experiments pertaining to pain (Barber & Cooper, 1972; Brown, Fader, & Barber, 1973; Chaves & Barber, in press), we derived the following hypothesis: subjects who are able to tolerate pain-producing stimulation are usually carrying out a specific "cognitive strategy"; for instance, they are purposively thinking of other things or they are thinking and imagining that the stimulated body part is made of rubber, has been injected with Novocain, or in some other way is numb and insensitive. We shall test this hypothesis in further research. Also, as part of our research in this area, we are at present beginning to develop methods that might be useful in teaching individuals to tolerate pain. Our preliminary work along these lines is described in the second part of this chapter.

AMNESIA

It has been commonly assumed that the "deeper" an individual is in "hypnotic trance" the more likely he is to forget the events when he is given suggestions for amnesia (cf. Wolberg, 1972, p. 152). From the cognitive-behavioral point of view, we can offer alternative conceptions of suggested amnesia. For instance, one alternative conception postulates that, when given suggestions to forget everything that occurred, a hypnotic subject and also a control subject who has positive attitudes, motivations, and expectancies toward the test situation does not let himself think about the events. This alternative conception is more harmonious than the "hypnotic trance" conception with five studies which showed that suggestions to forget what occurred are as effective with control subjects as with subjects who are said to be hypnotized (Barber & Calverley, 1966b; Norris, 1971; Spanos & Ham, 1973; Thorne, 1967, 1969; Thorne & Hall, 1969).

The alternative conception also receives some support from interviews that were conducted in a series of studies (Barber & Calverley, 1962; Blum, 1961; Hilgard, 1965; White, 1941). In these interviews, the subjects who had accepted the suggestion to forget the events commonly referred to their amnesia as follows:

"I haven't any inclination to go back over it"; "My mind doesn't want to think"; "I could remember it without being able to say it. Something inside me said 'You know what it is all the time.' I partly knew and partly didn't" (White, 1941).

". . . I know it but I can't think about it—I know what it is but I just kind of stop myself before I think of it" (Blum, 1961, p. 162).

"I put them out of my mind by thinking of [other things] "; "I grouped the tasks together as 'a group' to be forgotten"; "I just kept saying 'forget' to myself" (Barber & Calverley, 1962, p. 377).

Hilgard (1965) has summarized his data on this topic as follows:

We have tried to get subjects to tell us what amnesia is like. Often they reply sensibly enough that they have the helpless feeling that one has when trying to think of a name that doesn't come, but there are many variations. Some "see" the activities but cannot put them into words; others find that they do not want to make the effort to recall. Many report the "almost" recall, in which they know vaguely that something is there, just about ready to emerge into open recall [pp. 180-181].

Some of the cognitive processes that seem to be involved here have been conceptualized by Pattie (1965b) as "an attempt to occupy oneself with other things than an effort to recall" and by Rosenberg (1959) as a "motivated inattention" and a "vigorous suppression" of the events that are to be forgotten. These kinds of cognitive processes may not be as difficult as they appear. For instance, if the reader tells himself emphatically that he does not remember what he was doing yesterday at 2:30 p.m., he will recall the events only if he purposively makes the effort to think back. If he keeps his attention on the present and does not make the effort to think back, he can truthfully state and can have the feeling that he does not remember what he was doing yesterday at 2:30 p.m.

Although suggested amnesia at times seems to refer to a motivated unwillingness to think back to the events, it also at times seems to involve somewhat different cognitive processes. For instance, it may involve goal-directed imagining—that is, imagining a situation which, if it actually occurred, would tend to produce an inability to recall the material. In a recent study (Spanos & Ham, 1973), which we mentioned in Chapter 6, hypnotic subjects and also task motivated subjects whose eyes were closed were given a suggestion for selective amnesia—to forget the number 4. Most of the subjects who passed the suggestion seemed to engage in goal-directed imagining; for instance, a typical subject testified that she first visualized the numbers 1 to 10 on a blackboard and then visualized that the number 4 was erased. The hypnotic and task motivated subjects did not differ from one another either in the degree to which they reported forgetting or in their tendency to report goal-directed imagining.

Further research is needed to delineate more precisely the specific cognitive processes that are involved in suggested amnesia. We believe that when the processes are delineated, they will be within the range of normal human capabilities—it will not be necessary to postulate that a person carries out the cognitive processes more proficiently when he is in a "hypnotic trance."

CONTROL OF DREAMING

In a series of studies (Barber & Hahn, 1966; Stoyva, 1961; Tart, 1963; 1964; Tart & Dick, 1970) subjects were exposed to a hypnotic induction procedure and then were given suggestions to dream that night about a specified topic. The subjects were awakened at night during Stage 1 sleep, when the electroencephalogram and rapid eye movements indicated that they were dreaming. In some of the studies, the subjects were also awakened at times during Stages 2, 3, or 4 of sleep. When awakened during the night, the subjects reported what was passing through their minds or what they were dreaming. In each of the studies, the suggestions to dream at night on a specified topic were effective in producing some dream reports that pertained to the suggested topic.

The studies by Barber and Hahn (1966) and by Stoyva (1961) also included control subjects who were not exposed to a hypnotic induction procedure but who were given the suggestion to dream at night on the specified topic. In both studies, the nocturnal dreams were affected by suggestions given to control subjects. In the study by Barber and Hahn, the control subjects were generally as responsive as the hypnotic subjects to the suggestion to dream at night on a selected topic. In the study by Stoyva, the hypnotic subjects were given emphatic suggestions to dream at night on a specified topic, whereas the control subjects were given the suggestions lackadaisically in a "by the way" manner; in this case, the hypnotic subjects were more responsive to the suggestions than the control subjects.

The studies mentioned above suggest methods that might be used by individuals to control their own nocturnal dreams. For instance, in the Barber and Hahn (1966) study, a potent effect on dreams was obtained when the control subjects were told, immediately before they went to bed, to try to think about and to dream about the specified topic continuously throughout the night. How did these suggestions alter the contents of the nocturnal dreams? A provisional answer to this question is provided by the following two facts: (a) Thought processes do not stop when we are asleep. In fact, we continue to think, in a loose fashion, while we are asleep; these mental processes that occur during sleep are related to those that went on during the day and also to those that went on immediately before sleep onset (Foulkes, 1966). (b) The dreams that occur during sleep "do not arise *sui generis* as psychologically isolated mental productions but emerge as the most vivid and memorable part of a larger fabric of interwoven mental activity during sleep" (Rechtschaffen, Vogel, & Shaikun, 1963).

With the above two facts in mind, we can postulate that the suggestions to try to think and dream about a specified topic affected the contents of the nocturnal dreams as follows: (a) The subjects tried to focus their thoughts on the specified topic while they were falling asleep and also at other times during the night when they could voluntarily control their thoughts. (b) The mental processes that occurred during sleep were related to those that were present when the subject was falling asleep. (c) The contents of the nocturnal dreams were related to the mental activity that was occurring during the preceding period of sleep. These postulates suggest that we should be able to influence the contents of our nocturnal dreams by purposively thinking about a specific topic during the period that immediately precedes sleep and also at other times during the night when we can voluntarily control our thoughts.

Tart (1963) also presented data suggesting the possibility that suggestions given to subjects immediately before going to bed at night may be effective at times in inducing the subjects to awaken at the beginning of their dreams, to awaken at the end of their dreams, and, possibly, to increase the amount of time they spend dreaming during the night. Tart (1970) has also provided experimental data indicating that some individuals may be able to awaken in the morning at a time they preselected before going to bed at night.

Further studies are needed to expand the findings discussed above. It appears that intensive work in this area may be able to specify precise methods that individuals can use to influence the contents of their dreams, to acquire the ability to awaken at the beginning or at the end of their dreams, to increase the amount of time they dream during the night, and to awaken in the morning at a preselected time.

CONTROL OF SKIN TEMPERATURE

Studies by Harano et al, (1965) and by Schultz (1926), which were summarized in Chapter 6 of this text, indicate that we have the potential to produce localized changes in skin temperature. Along similar lines, Menzies (1941) found that some individuals show localized vasodilation (with a rise in skin temperature) when recalling previous experiences involving warmth of the limb and localized vasoconstriction (with a drop in skin temperature) when recalling experiences involving cold. In an earlier study, Hadfield (1920) also demonstrated that localized changes in skin temperature could be produced by suggestions. In this case, the subject had exercised vigorously before the experiment and the temperature of both hands had reached 95° F. It was then suggested to the subject that the right hand was becoming cold. Within half an hour, the temperature of the right palm fell to 68°, while the temperature of the left palm remained at 94°. When next given the suggestion that the right hand was becoming warm, the temperature of the hand rose within 20 minutes to 94°. Although this subject had previously participated in hypnotic experiments, Hadfield insisted that he did not "hypnotize" her during this experiment and that the temperature alterations occurred when the subject was entirely in the "waking condition."

Two studies (Green, Ferguson, Green, & Walters, 1970; Wenger & Bagchi, 1961) have demonstrated that some trained yogis are able to produce localized changes in skin temperature. In the case presented by Wenger and Bagchi, the yogi could produce perspiration on his forehead within ten minutes after he began concentrating. The authors provided the following background data:

> This man had spent part of two winters in caves in the Himalayas. During such periods, usually alone and unclad except for an animal skin, much of his time was spent in meditation. . . . The cold distracted him, and his teacher advised him to concentrate on *warmth* and to visualize himself in extremely high temperature situations. . . . He reported gradual success *after about six months of practice*. Later he

found that in a moderate climate the same practices produced not only increased sensations of warmth but perspiration [p. 313].

More recently, Zimbardo, Maslach, and Marshall (1970) presented experimental data showing that some individuals can exercise cognitive control over skin temperature. Three subjects were used who had received an extensive period of training in "hypnosis"—that is, who had received extensive training in learning to relax deeply, to concentrate, to imagine vividly, and to dissociate themselves from specified stimuli. In the experimental session, each subject was first exposed to a hypnotic induction procedure that focused on deep relaxation. Each subject was then asked to make one hand hot and the other cold; several images were suggested that could be useful in producing these effects. The subject was also encouraged to give himself suggestions and to generate his own imagery. All three subjects were able to lower the temperature of one hand by about $2°$ to $7°$ F. Two of the three subjects were able to raise the temperature of the other hand by about $2°$ F. The increases and decreases in skin temperature were typically associated with imaginings along the following lines: The subject imagined that one hand was in a bucket of ice water while the other hand was under a heat lamp, or the subject imagined that one hand was becoming red with anger while the other was becoming white with fear. Subjects in a comparison group, who had not received the extensive period of training in "hypnosis" (in relaxing, concentrating, imagining, etc.) and who were not exposed to a hypnotic induction procedure, were unable to produce a significant alteration in the temperature of the hands.

The data summarized above and other recent data (Roberts, Kewman, & Macdonald, 1973) suggest the possibility that many individuals might be able to produce localized changes in the temperature of their skin after they have received training in thinking and imagining that the skin is cold or warm. We might tentatively offer the hypothesis that the drop in skin temperature is mediated by variables such as the following: When vividly imagining that a limb is exposed to cold, the subject may tend to tense the muscles in the limb; contraction of the muscles tends to produce vasoconstriction; vasoconstriction, in turn, produces the drop in skin temperature. We might also tentatively hypothesize that the mediating variables producing a rise in skin temperature may involve the following: When a subject becomes involved in imagining that a limb is exposed to warmth, he tends to relax the muscles in the limb; muscular relaxation tends to produce vasodilation; vasodilation, in turn, produces the rise in skin temperature. We venture to predict that in the near future the mediating mechanisms will be delineated and direct methods for training individuals to manifest temperature control will be developed.

IMPROVING NEARSIGHTED VISION

Four carefully conducted investigations (Graham & Leibowitz, 1972; Harwood, 1970, 1971; Kelley, 1958) have demonstrated that visual acuity in myopic individuals can be heightened by suggestions to imagine something pleasant and by suggestions to relax the muscles around the eyes.

Fourteen myopic individuals participated in Kelley's (1958) study. The subjects were first tested for "hypnotizability." Seven were rated as poor hypnotic subjects and the other seven were rated as fair or good hypnotic subjects. In the experimental sessions, the poor hypnotic subjects were not exposed to a hypnotic induction procedure; instead, they were given suggestions for improved visual acuity under a control condition. The fair and good hypnotic subjects were exposed to a hypnotic induction procedure and then given the same suggestions for improved vision. The subjects participated in from one to three experimental sessions. Three types of suggestions were used to improve visual acuity. (a) It was suggested that, when the subject opened his eyes, he would look at the material on the vision-testing chart with an attitude of relaxed interest and effortlessness, without making any particular effort to see. (b) The experimenter asked the subject to imagine a series of pleasant scenes; he then suggested to the subject that, when he opened his eyes and looked at the chart, he would continue to maintain the feeling that he had developed while imagining the pleasant scenes. (c) It was suggested that the subject would feel as if he were looking over great distances when he looked at the chart. Although each type of suggestion was effective wtih some subjects, the suggestion to imagine pleasant scenes was the most effective and was used most often. Twelve of the 14 subjects showed improved visual acuity for distant objects. The control group improved as much as the hypnotic group. The overall average improvement of both groups was equivalent to the differences between 20/50 and 20/20 acuity.

In a recent investigation, Graham and Leibowitz (1972) suggested to myopic subjects that they would relax the muscles around and behind the eyes. Each subject participated in three experimental sessions conducted at weekly intervals. About half of the myopic subjects were always given the suggestions to relax the eyes immediately after they had been exposed to a hypnotic induction procedure and the other myopic subjects, used as controls, were always given the same suggestions without a preceding hypnotic induction. At the end of each session, each subject was told to practice relaxing his eyes at home. The procedures were effective in producing a small but statistically significant improvement in visual acuity in most of the myopic subjects. The control group improved as much as the hypnotic group. The improvement in visual acuity was greater for the more myopic subjects and also for those subjects who had obtained higher scores on the Barber Suggestibility Scale.

Did the subjects participating in the Graham and Leibowitz investigation maintain their improved visual acuity outside of the experimental setting? The subjects were tested twice outside of the experimental setting by an optometrist —before they participated in the experimental sessions and soon after the sessions were completed. In a few of the hypnotic subjects (especially those who originally showed the greatest degree of myopia), the improved visual acuity that was produced in the experimental setting was also present when they were tested by the optometrist soon after the experimental sessions were completed.

Graham and Leibowitz (1972) also conducted another study with five myopic subjects. This study aimed at determining the mechanisms underlying the improved visual acuity that is produced by suggestions. Using a recently developed technique that involves a laser, Graham and Leibowitz showed that the improved acuity was *not* due to changes in the refractive power of the eye. Whether the improvement was due to more adequate utilization of perceptual cues available in the test situation or to other factors remains to be determined.

The studies summarized above have been replicated and extended by Harwood (1970,1971). He also used a hypnotic group and a control group. The hypnotic group was comprised of three selected good hypnotic subjects who were exposed to a hypnotic induction procedure. The control group was comprised of three selected poor hypnotic subjects who had been taught to relax by utilizing a variant of Jacobson's progressive relaxation technique. During the experiments, the hypnotic subjects and also the control subjects were given suggestions that they could deal with the visual tasks with confidence, with a relaxed mind, and with relaxed and calm eyes. The suggestions were effective in producing improved visual acuity in all of the hypnotic subjects and in all of the control subjects. In general, the subjects showed an enhancement of visual acuity of about 15%. This small degree of improvement appeared to be due to increased motivation and concentration and to the reduction of the apprehension that is usually present when visual acuity is measured. However, the same subjects who showed a small improvement also at times showed a marked improvement in which they could perceive targets that were half the size of those they could perceive previously. The impressive changes in visual acuity may have been due to "the shifting of the perceptual mechanism to a different set of clues for the discovery of the essential information which leads to the identification of the target" (Harwood, 1970).

The studies summarized above suggest the possibility that nearsighted individuals may set their standards for visual performance lower than necessary. As Graham and Leibowitz (1972) pointed out, "Through failure to see distant objects as clearly as desired, he [the nearsighted person] may become progressively more dependent upon the corrective lenses and no longer try to exceed the internal standard" (p. 184). However, it appears that specific kinds of suggestions—e.g., suggestions to imagine pleasant scenes or suggestions to relax the eye muscles—are effective in inducing a substantial proportion of myopic individuals to utilize their normally-unused potential. Further studies in this area are needed to delineate more precisely the kinds of instructions and suggestions that are the most effective and the physiological mechanisms that are involved in improving visual acuity in myopic individuals.

CONTROL OF ALLERGIES

There is evidence to indicate that some types of allergic responses can be brought under cognitive control. Ikemi and Nakagawa (1962) worked with 13 subjects who were very allergic to the leaves of two common poisonous trees found in Japan (the lacquer tree and the wax tree). Five of the subjects were exposed to a hypnotic induction procedure and eight subjects were assigned to a control treatment. (The hypnotic subjects kept their eyes closed and the control subjects were blindfolded.) All subjects were given the suggestion that they were being touched with the leaves of a harmless tree (the chestnut tree) while they were actually touched with the leaves of the allergy-producing trees. When thus given the suggestion that the leaves were harmless, four of the five subjects under the hypnotic treatment and seven of the eight under the control treatment did not manifest the expected allergic response. Next, the harmless chestnut leaves were applied to the alternate arm while the subject received the suggestion that he was being touched by the leaves from one of the allergy-producing trees. In this case, the harmless leaves gave rise to a slight to marked degree of dermatitis —for example, flushing, erythema, papules—in all hypnotic subjects and in all control subjects. In brief, the results presented by Ikemi and Nakagawa strongly indicated that in allergic individuals (a) suggestions that an allergic substance is harmless are sufficient to inhibit an allergic response, (b) suggestions that a harmless substance is an allergic substance are sufficient to elicit some aspects of an allergic response, and (c) formal hypnotic induction procedures are irrelevant in eliciting these effects. Further studies in this area might enhance our understanding of psychosomatic processes and of human potentialities.

RECAPITULATION

Let us restate a theme underlying the foregoing discussion. The traditional viewpoint seems to assume that a "special state" (a "hypnotic trance," a "somnambulistic state," a "deep hypnotic state," etc.) is needed to produce many of the important phenomena that are associated with suggestions such as control of pain, amnesia, control of dreaming, control of skin temperature, enhanced visual acuity, and inhibition of allergic responses. Our viewpoint, which regards the concept of *hypnotic trance* as misleading, allows for a broader conception of the capabilities and potentialities of normal human beings. Our viewpoint postulates that (a) the phenomena are elicited when an individual thinks and imagines with the themes that are suggested and (b) a large proportion of individuals have the potential to think and imagine with the themes of suggestions. However, (c) the potential often remains dormant until the individual has positive attitudes, motivations, and expectancies toward the situation. Methods that might prove useful for producing the necessary attitudes, motivations, and expectancies and that might also directly help individuals to think and imagine with the themes of suggestions are discussed in the next section.

TRAINING IN HUMAN POTENTIALITIES

Since 1969, while conducting group workshops and also while working with a small number of individual subjects, one of the authors (T.X.B.) has been developing a course that we have labeled *Training in Human Potentialities*. Although at the present time the course has not been finalized and only some parts of the course have been evaluated experimentally (Chaves & Barber, in press; Comins, Fullam, & Barber, 1973), there are two reasons for our belief that it is worthwhile to outline it here: (a) the outline should illustrate in a concrete manner how some of the principles developed in this text can be applied and (b) other investigators may see the procedures as useful and may proceed to evaluate them experimentally.[1] We shall describe the course as a first-person report, as it is seen by the experimenter (T.X.B.).

Defining the Situation

I typically define the situation as one in which the subject will learn to fulfill his own potentialities. I tell the subject that I can help him learn how to focus his thoughts, how to recall useful material by vividly imagining a previous situation, how to improve his learning proficiency, how to control pain, and how to control his bodily processes by first learning to control his mental processes. I emphasize to the subject that the training he receives in the experimental situation should prove useful in his daily life.

Learning to Control Pain

Although I can begin the training course in various ways, I usually begin by trying to teach the subject how to control pain. I tell him that he will first learn to tolerate a normally painful stimulus and not be bothered by it at all. I also explain to him that the learning will be useful in a wide variety of situations in which he normally experiences pain. For instance, I might state:

> It should be useful not only in overcoming the pains and discomforts of daily life but also in dentistry and [for female subjects] during childbirth. Once you have learned how to control pain, you may be able to transfer or extrapolate what you have learned to other situations in your life in which anxiety, distress, or fear are present.

I then expose the subject for a period of one minute to the Forgione-Barber (1971) pain stimulator, which brings a weight to bear on the bony part of a finger. Next, I tell the subject that he can control the pain produced by the weight by keeping his mind on other things during the stimulation and also by imagining vividly that the stimulated finger is dull, numb, or insensitive.

Next, I model for the subject. I show him how I can control pain by utilizing the two techniques mentioned above. I place the weight on my own finger and then I state, "I am going to think of other things. I am not going to let myself think of the heavy weight on my finger." While the weight remains on my finger, I verbalize some of the things I am thinking about; for example: "I am thinking back to last summer when I was on the beach. . . . I am sitting on the hot sand. . . . The sun is hot but pleasant. . . . As I enter the water, I find it is comfortably cool. . . . In the distance I see an airplane slowly moving overhead. . . ." I continue for several minutes to verbalize some of the things I am thinking and visualizing, while the weight remains on my finger and I show no signs of pain or distress.

I then state, "I will now try to think of the finger as numb and insensitive. . . . I am imagining that Novocain has been injected into the finger. . . . I am thinking of the Novocain spreading slowly throughout the finger and it is becoming dull, numb, like a piece of rubber. . . . I am imagining that the finger is just a piece of matter—a lump of matter without feelings or sensations. . . ." For several minutes I continue imagining numbness and insensitivity and I verbalize my thoughts aloud without showing signs of pain or distress.

Finally, I remove the weight from my finger and I tell the subject that he can control pain by using the same procedures. I ask him to try, to the best of his ability, to think and imagine in the way I have just demonstrated. The heavy weight is then placed on the subject's finger and he practices carrying out the processes of trying to think of other things and then trying to imagine that the finger has become insensitive. Although some subjects find it difficult to think and imagine in this way, other subjects are able to do it rather easily and they succeed in tolerating the pain-producing stimulus.

In the further development of this course, I hope to delineate other techniques that subjects can use to control pain. Some techniques that might prove useful include thinking and imagining that the stimulated body part is just a "thing" that is not actually part of oneself, and thinking of the sensations not as "pain" but as a variety of unusual sensations with their own unique properties. Also, in further development of the course, I expect to give subjects additional practice in tolerating pain produced by other kinds of stimuli—for instance, pain produced by immersion of a limb in ice water and pain produced by blocking off the blood supply to an arm by means of a tourniquet. When a subject has learned to control pain in the laboratory, I shall attempt to determine if his learning can be transferred to a situation outside the laboratory. For instance, I shall ask the subject to try to undergo his next dental appointment without Novocain and to try to utilize what he has learned in the laboratory—to try to think of other things during the dentistry or to try to imagine that Novocain has been injected and that his teeth and gums have become insensitive. As I develop the training course, I also hope to find methods that subjects can use to transfer what they have learned to other situations in their daily lives that involve anxiety or pain.

Learning to Experience a Variety of Phenomena

Although I typically begin the course by trying to teach the subject to tolerate pain, I can also begin in other ways—for example, by first trying to teach the subject how to experience a variety of effects that have been traditionally associated with suggestions and hypnotism.

In teaching the subject to experience a variety of interesting phenomena, I use procedures that are similar to those that were described above. I first tell the subject that he can fulfill his potentialities by learning to control his thinking and imagining. I then state that he will receive practice in focusing his thinking and imagining on the idea that one arm is very heavy and rigid, the other arm is very light and is rising, his body is rigid and immovable, he feels very thirsty, etc. I then model for the subject, verbalizing how I am experiencing one of these phenomena, such as arm heaviness and rigidity, by thinking and imagining that my arm is heavy and rigid. I may also explain to the subject that when I think and vividly imagine that my arm is rigid, the muscles of my arm naturally contract; the contraction of the muscles makes my arm feel heavy and rigid; then, by keeping my thoughts on the induced heaviness and rigidity, my arm can feel exceedingly heavy and rigid.

After the subject has attempted to carry out the same kind of cognitive processes, I interview him to determine to what extent he was able to concentrate on the idea of heaviness or rigidity. If the subject reports that negative thoughts intruded (for example, the thought that "My arm cannot become heavy and rigid"), I tell him to try it again while trying to imagine more vividly and that, if he concentrates on imagining, the negative thoughts will disappear.

The same procedures are used to teach the subject to experience other phenomena such as arm levitation, body immobility, thirst hallucination, amnesia, age regression, and relaxation. Let me describe how the general procedures are applied to the latter two phenomena—age regression and relaxation.

Experiencing Age Regression

I tell the subject that he can heighten his recall of earlier events by vividly imagining a past time. I also give several examples of how this technique is useful in daily life. For instance, I tell the subject that when he is taking an examination and he wishes to recall material that he learned previously, he can heighten his recall by imagining and clearly visualizing the concrete situation in which he originally learned the material. I then state:

> I will show you how to reexperience a past time. In a moment, I will close my eyes so that I can remove distractions. Then, I will tell myself that I am ten years of age and I will imagine and visualize that I am in the fourth grade classroom. I will then concentrate my thinking and imagining on the idea that I am ten years old and, when I succeed in concentrating my thinking and imagining around this idea, thoughts that I am an adult in an experimental situation will not arise. Once I begin clearly visualizing the fourth grade, I will let my imagination "move" and I will let myself "go with" the events that I imagine.

I then close my eyes. After a few minutes, I open them. I state that I felt I was ten years old, and I describe how I experienced myself, the teacher, and the students in the classroom.

I then tell the subject:

> In a minute I will ask you to close your eyes and to think back to the time you were ten years old. Imagine that you are sitting in the classroom. Concentrate your thinking and imagining on the idea that you are in the classroom; feel yourself in that situation, and then let your imagination "move." As you let the teacher, the students, and yourself interact and "come alive," thoughts about the present or thoughts about your being an adult in an experimental situation will disappear.

The subject is then given practice in experiencing himself as ten years old. Subsequently, he is given further practice in experiencing various other age levels.

Experiencing Relaxation

I introduce the training in relaxation by speaking to the subject along the following lines:

> Most individuals are so busy living their daily lives that they rarely, if ever, allow themselves to experience total relaxation. In fact, it is questionable whether most individuals know how to relax. This is unfortunate because the ability to relax completely is very useful in our daily lives. Once we have learned to relax, we are able to remain clam and at ease in many situations that normally produce anxiety or tension. For instance, many individuals become tense or anxious when they meet new people, when they are in a strange or new situation, and when they feel that they are being judged by others. Also, individuals who are alcoholics or who are obese or who cannot quit smoking become tense and anxious when they have not had alcohol or food or a cigarette for a period of time. Some individuals also have specific kinds of fears; for instance, fear of riding in an airplane, fear of heights, or fear of narrow spaces. If these individuals could learn how to relax, they could control their anxiety, tension, or fear. An important fact that has been emphasized by behavior therapists is that anxiety and tension are incompatible with physical and mental relaxation. If a person lets himself relax, he can control or block the anxiety, tension, or fear. In fact, many of the useful effects that are attributed to yoga,

hypnosis, Zen, and transcendental meditation appear to be due to the relaxation that is produced by each of these techniques.

I next state that I will now model for the subject, showing him how to relax. I introduce the modeling demonstration as follows:

> I will now show you how to relax. To get rid of distractions, I will first close my eyes. Then I will think to myself that I am becoming very relaxed. I will tell myself that my arms are relaxing, my legs are relaxing, my eyes are relaxing, all parts of my body are relaxing. I will then imagine that I am floating on a soft cloud and that my body feels very, very relaxed. I will continue telling myself that I am completely relaxed and I will imagine scenes, such as floating softly on smooth water, which will make me feel more and more relaxed.

I then model for the subject, demonstrating how to relax. After a few minutes, I open my eyes, report what I was thinking and imagining during the period of relaxation, and then ask the subject to try relaxing in the same way. I may give the subject several practice trials during the session, asking him to relax for longer and longer periods of time. Before the subject leaves, I usually ask him to continue practicing the relaxation technique at home and to try to use what he has learned about relaxation in his daily life whenever he begins to feel anxious or tense.

Experimental Evaluation

The effectiveness of parts of the above course of training have been evaluated experimentally. In one recent experiment (Comins, Fullam, & Barber 1973), the experimenter modeled for one group of subjects, showing them (a) how he thought and imagined those things that he suggested aloud to himself (arm heaviness, arm levitation, hand clasp, and thirst "hallucination") and (b) how he, consequently, experienced an involuntary lowering and rising of his arm, an inability to unclasp his hands, and extreme thirst. The subjects who had observed the experimenter responding to test suggestions were then tested on the Barber Suggestibility Scale. Their scores on the scale were compared with the scores of two random groups of subjects: a control group that had not received any instructions and a hypnotic induction group that had been exposed to repeated suggestions of relaxation, drowsiness, and hypnotic sleep. Subjects who had observed the experimenter model were markedly more responsive than the control subjects to the test suggestions of the Barber Suggestibility Scale and they were as responsive as the subjects who had been exposed to the standardized hypnotic induction procedure.

In a second evaluative study (Chaves & Barber, in press), 120 subjects were first exposed to a pain pretest (a heavy weight was applied to a finger for two minutes). Before receiving the pain stimulus a second time (posttest), some of the subjects were told to imagine pleasant events during the pain stimulation, others were told to imagine that the finger was insensitive, and the remaining subjects were used as controls. With regard to the subjects who were told to imagine, half were and half were not exposed to experimenter modeling. Those who were exposed to experimenter modeling observed how the experimenter could tolerate the pain when he imagined pleasant events or imagined that the finger was insensitive. Overall, subjects who were told to imagine pleasant events or to imagine that the finger was insensitive reported less pain than the control subjects. Also, the experimenter modeling procedure was effective in producing a further reduction in pain in subjects who reported a high level of pain during the pretest and who were asked to imagine pleasant events during the posttest.

Although the above two studies evaluated the effects of the experimenter modeling procedure, they did not define the situation to the subjects as one in which they could learn to fulfill their potentialities. Further studies are planned to test the separate and combined effects of (a) defining the situation as training in human potentialities and (b) experimenter modeling.

SUMMARY

The cognitive-behavioral viewpoint presented in this text suggests a broadened conception of human capabilities and potentialities. A wide range of experiences that have been traditionally associated with a special condition (a "hypnotic trance") are viewed as potentially within the repertoire of most normal individuals. Data were presented in the chapter to support the contention that a special state is not necessary for individuals to control pain, to experience amnesia, to influence the contents of their nocturnal dreams, to exert localized control over their skin temperature, to increase their visual acuity, and to control their allergic responses.

The last part of the chapter outlined a course, now being developed, that aims to teach individuals how to control pain and how to experience age regression, relaxation, arm levitation, limb rigidity, and other useful or interesting phenomena. The course is defined to the subject as *Training in Human Potentialities*. A unique feature of the course is that the *experimenter models* for the subject. The experimenter demonstrates how he himself can think and imagine that his finger is insensitive, that he is a child, that he is floating on a cloud, and, consequently, that he can control pain, can experience age regression, can relax, etc. After the experimenter demonstrates how he himself goes about having each experience, the subject is asked to try to think and imagine in the same way and is given practice in having the experience. Two recent experimental studies indicated that the experimenter modeling procedure is a useful technique for teaching subjects how to respond to suggestions. Further studies are planned that will also evaluate the effectiveness of defining the situation to the subjects as "training in human potentialities."

NOTES

[1] Diamond (1972), Kinney (1969), and Sachs (1971) have also recently presented methods for training hypnotic subjects to become more responsive to test suggestions. The training procedures we are presenting in this section differ in several important respects and were developed independently from those presented by Diamond, Kinney, and Sachs. However, the methods we have been using also have several features in common with those developed by other investigators. These various methods for training subjects will be discussed together in Chapter 11.

Where Do We Go From Here?

Science is not a static enterprise. It involves the continual reexamination of established phenomena and the discovery of new phenomena. It also involves the continual revision and extension of theories that are used to explain the phenomena.

The cognitive-behavioral theory presented in this text will certainly change in numerous respects as new data become available. Some aspects of the theory will be shown to be either misleading or useless and will be discarded. Other aspects may guide investigators toward useful research that gives rise to new insights. Where will the theory take us? What are the limitations of the theory? What kind of research can the theory generate that will further clarify the phenomena associated wtih hypnotism? In this chapter, these general questions will be translated into the following four specific questions: (a) How can we clarify the role of the complex conglomerate of variables that comprise an induction procedure? (b) How can we delineate experimentally the relevance of subjects' attitudes, motivations, and expectancies? (c) How can we proceed to gain a deeper understanding of the processes involved in thinking and imagining with the themes of the suggestions? Finally, (d) how can the area of hypnotism be integrated with other aspects of psychology?

VARIABLES IN INDUCTION PROCEDURES

In Chapter 3, we described eight variables in induction procedures that seem to influence the subject's response. However, we do not know whether the variables are additive and what combination of variables produce the maximum effect. For instance, we simply cannot say whether a maximum level of responsiveness is obtained when the subject is exposed to all eight variables or whether only three or four of the variables are sufficient to elicit maximum responsiveness.

Furthermore, we need more information about each of the eight variables taken alone. For instance, much more work is needed to clarify the effects of such vocal qualities of suggestions as inflections, stresses, pauses, rate of delivery, and tone of voice. Similarly, we need to iron out the effects of simply keeping the eyes closed for a period of time. It may be that keeping the eyes closed is sufficient to enhance responsiveness to some test suggestions—for instance, suggestions of age regression. Simply keeping the eyes closed for a period of time may also give rise to some of the experiences that have been traditionally associated with hypnotism—for example, feeling as if one's body is very small or as if one's head is very large.

Role of Relaxation-Sleep-Hypnosis Suggestions

Hypnotists expose their subjects to many kinds of suggestions. These include relaxation-sleep-hypnosis suggestions and also test suggestions for arm rigidity, analgesia, age regression, and amnesia. The repeated suggestions for relaxation, drowsiness, sleep, and hypnosis are given at the beginning of the session because it is presumed that they produce the "hypnotic trance" that is thought to be essential for obtaining a high level of responsiveness to test suggestions. However, it is possible to view the relaxation-sleep-hypnosis suggestions as another set of test suggestions to which the subject may or may not respond.

If relaxation-sleep-hypnosis suggestions are viewed primarily as another set of test suggestions, one might predict the following: correlations between response to relaxation-sleep-hypnosis suggestions and response to other types of test suggestions will be equally high regardless of whether the relaxation-sleep-hypnosis suggestions are given at the beginning or at the end of the session. For instance, one might predict that a correlation of, say, +0.70 will be obtained between response to relaxation-sleep-hypnosis suggestions and response to a test suggestion for arm rigidity when the relaxation-sleep-hypnosis suggestions *precede* the arm rigidity suggestion and also when they are given *after* the arm rigidity suggestion.[1] We believe that faster progress can be made in this area by testing this and similar kinds of hypotheses that derive from the notion that relaxation-sleep-hypnosis suggestions are primarily another set of test suggestions instead of a very special set of suggestions that produce a special state.

Role of the Hypnotist

We have little information about the effects on the subject's responsiveness of the hypnotist's personal characteristics such as age, sex, race, ethnicity, dominance, friendliness, and prestige (Balaschak, Blocker, Rossiter, & Perin, 1972; Cronin, Spanos, & Barber, 1971; Greenberg & Land, 1971; Weitzenhoffer & Weitzenhoffer, 1958). Also, we do not know to what extent the subject's performance is related to the hypnotist's conceptions of hypnotism: for example, whether he views hypnotism as a situation in which his need for power can be exercised or as one that is erotically-tinged or as an implicit sexual encounter. If the hypnotist views the situation in terms of power, he may use an authoritative tone of voice in administering his suggestions; if he sees it as erotically-tinged, he may use a seductive tone of voice; and his tone of voice may affect the subject's response (Barber & Calverley, 1964b).

We also need to look more closely at how the interpersonal relationship between the subject and the hypnotist affects the subject's performance. For instance, when a hypnotist reports that a "trained" subject was very responsive to suggestions, to what extent is he referring to a subject who, during the "training," developed a close relationship with him and, as a result of the relationship, was willing to oblige or to perform as requested (Barber, 1961a)?

ATTITUDES, MOTIVATIONS, AND EXPECTANCIES

The theory presented in this text has emphasized that the subject's responsiveness to test suggestions is in part mediated by his attitudes, motivations, and expectancies. This formulation needs to be delineated more precisely. Questions such as the following should be answered: Are all three factors—positive attitudes *and* positive motivations *and* positive expectancies—equally relevant for high response to test suggestions? How does a subject respond to suggestions if he has positive attitudes (if he generally views "hypnosis" or responding to suggestions as worthwhile or valuable) and positive motivation (if he *now* tries to be "hypnotized" or tries to experience those things that are suggested) but, at the same time, has a negative expectancy (if he believes that he himself cannot actually be "hypnotized" or have the experiences that are suggested)? A series of related questions are also important. For instance, how does a subject respond to test suggestions if he believes that he can be easily "hypnotized" (positive expectancy) but, at the same time, is fearful or has negative attitudes towards "hypnosis." Which of these three factors plays the most important role? How do they interrelate?

Of course, a major problem in this area is to find better methods for assessing the subject's attitudes, motivations, and expectancies prior to and also during the experiment. Social psychologists have developed a wide variety of direct and indirect techniques for measuring these kinds of variables, and some of these techniques could also be used in the area of hypnotism (Edwards, 1957; Kiesler, Collins, & Miller, 1969; Secord & Backman, 1964; Webb, Campbell, Schwartz, & Sechrest, 1966).

Much more work is also needed that focuses on each of these variables separately. For instance, let us look briefly at the kind of research that might clarify the role of the subjects' attitudes toward hypnotism. Many subjects who are asked to participate in hypnotic experiments appear to have at least partly negative attitudes. They seem to view hypnotism as a situation in which they will be brought under the control of another person or as one in which they will be shown to be gullible. These negative attitudes, in turn, appear to produce negative motivations and a low level of responsiveness. Further studies are needed that attempt to change subjects' attitudes toward hypnotism. Further studies are also needed that attempt to define responsiveness to test suggestions in a more favorable light—for instance, as "training in human potentialities." We predict that as better and better techniques are developed for removing negative attitudes, our subject population will be found to be more and more responsive to test suggestions.

THINKING AND IMAGINING WITH THE THEMES OF THE SUGGESTIONS

Our cognitive-behavioral theory postulates that responsiveness to test suggestions is related to the extent to which the subject thinks and imagines with the themes of the suggestions. Although we believe this formulation is useful, it needs to be extended to account for the fact that some test suggestions are passed by almost all subjects, while others are failed by almost all subjects. We believe that there are at least two major reasons why some test suggestions are easy and others are difficult to pass. (a) Some test suggestions, but not others, provide a "cognitive strategy," that is, they tell the subject how to think and imagine in order to experience that which is suggested. (b) When exposed to some test suggestions, but not others, the subject is at the same time exposed to sensory feedback or other kinds of information that contradict what he is supposed to experience. Let us examine each of these factors separately.

Cognitive Strategies

All test suggestions that have been historically associated with hypnotism inform the subject as to the overt behaviors and subjective experiences that are expected to occur. For instance, a test suggestion for arm levitation informs the subject that his arm is to rise upwards and he is to have the experience that the arm rose involuntarily—"by itself." Similarly, a test suggestion for arm rigidity informs the subject that his arm is to become rigid "by itself" and he is to have the experience that he is unable to bend it.

Although all test suggestions inform the subject that a specific behavior is to occur, only some test suggestions provide the subject with a method—a cognitive strategy—that he can use to carry out the behavior while perceiving it as occurring without his active volition. Quite often the cognitive strategy that is provided asks the subject to carry out goal-directed imagining (that is, to imagine a specific situation which, if it were the actual state of affairs, would tend to produce the behavior and experience that are being suggested). For instance, a suggestion for arm levitation might ask the subject to imagine a large helium-filled balloon tied to the wrist which is raising the arm.

Some test suggestions, however, do not provide the subject with a cognitive strategy that can help him experience the suggested effect. For instance, suggestions for amnesia clearly inform the subject about what he is to forget, but usually tell him little or nothing about how he is to go about forgetting.

In brief, test suggestions differ in the extent to which they provide an explicit cognitive strategy for performing the desired behavior while, at the same time, experiencing it as occurring involuntarily. Thus, to pass some test suggestions, a subject must *implement* a cognitive strategy that is provided by the wording of the suggestion, whereas, to pass another test suggestion, the subject must both *devise* and *implement* a cognitive strategy. These considerations suggest the hypothesis that test suggestions are easier, are experienced by a greater number of subjects, when they provide an explicit cognitive strategy for the subjects to follow. Let us examine two studies that bear on the validity of this hypothesis.

Data pertaining to cognitive strategies. A study by Spanos and Barber (1972) supports the hypothesis that responses to test suggestions can be more easily experienced as occurring involuntarily when the wording of the suggestion provides the subject with an explicit cognitive strategy. In this study, three randomized groups of subjects who had been exposed to a standardized hypnotic induction procedure were given suggestions for arm levitation. The suggestions given to one group included an explicit cognitive strategy for experiencing the arm rising as occurring "by itself"—that is, the subjects were told explicitly to imagine a helium-filled balloon tied to the wrist that was pulling the arm up. The suggestion given to the second group was worded as follows: "Your arm is beginning to rise. It's rising, going up and up. ..." The suggestion given to the third group was worded in this way: "Imagine your arm is beginning to rise. Imagine it's rising, going up and up. ..." It should be noted that the latter two suggestions also implied that the arm levitation was to be experienced as occurring involuntarily, but these suggestions did not include an explicit cognitive strategy for experiencing the arm rising as occurring "by itself." Subjects given the suggestion that provided an explicit cognitive strategy (to imagine a balloon that was pulling the arm up) more often had the experience that the arm was rising involuntarily ("by itself") than those given the suggestions that did not provide an explicit cognitive strategy.

Another team of investigators (Coe, Allen, Krug, & Wurzmann, 1972) used a different procedure to evaluate the importance of goal-directed imagining as a type of cognitive strategy. These investigators counted the number of words in a series of standardized test suggestions that directed the subject to imagine specific events that were related to the suggested effect. The test suggestions were then ordered along a continuum extending from those that did not contain any words indicating that the subject should engage in goal-directed imagining to those that were highly explicit in specifying the type of goal-directed imagining that was to be carried out. Significant positive correlations were obtained between the following variables: (a) the number of words in a suggestion that encouraged goal-directed imagining and the subject's tendency to carry out goal-directed imagining, (b) the number of words in a suggestion that encouraged goal-directed imagining and the likelihood that the test suggestion was passed, and (c) the number of times that the subjects reported goal-directed imagining and their responsiveness to the test suggestions.

Taken together, the two studies summarized above indicate that the way suggestions are worded plays an important role in determining whether they are easy or difficult to pass. More specifically, these studies indicate that suggested effects can be experienced more readily if the suggestions explicitly provide the subject with a cognitive strategy—if they inform him how he is to think and imagine in order to have the suggested experience.

The studies summarized above also suggest a two-part research program that might increase our understanding of hypnotism. The first part of the program would aim to discover the cognitive strategies that subjects use to pass test suggestions. In the second part of the program, the cognitive strategies would be taught to subjects in order to enhance their responsiveness to test suggestions. We shall now illustrate how this research program could be applied, using a suggestion for selective amnesia as our example.

Proposed research on cognitive strategies. As was pointed out earlier, test suggestions for amnesia always inform the subject about what to forget but usually do not tell him how to go about forgetting. Thus, one step in carrying out a research program in this area would involve discovering the cognitive strategies that are used by subjects to pass suggestions for amnesia. The most direct method for discovering such cognitive strategies is to ask subjects to give detailed descriptions of their experiences. For instance, in two recent studies (Spanos, 1971; Spanos & Ham, 1973), interviews were conducted with subjects who had been given a difficult suggestion for selective amnesia—to forget the number 4. These studies indicated that subjects who report forgetting the number typically imagine a line of numbers in which the 4 is missing. The subjects often devised rather elaborate imaginings that led to the "disappearance" of the (imagined) number 4. For example, one subject imagined the number 4 disintegrating, another subject imagined that it was shot into space and out of view like a rocket ship, and a third subject imagined that a man pulled the number 4 out of line with a hook. These subjects also indicated that they did not experience themselves as actively trying to force the number 4 out of their consciousness. Instead, their reports indicated that they simply let themselves "go with" their imaginings and they were not concerned whether the contents of their imaginings were "real" occurrences.

Having delineated at least one cognitive strategy for forgetting a number, the next step in the proposed research program is to teach this strategy to other subjects and, thereby, to enhance their ability to pass the test suggestions. Studies aimed at teaching subjects how to forget a specific number have yet to be carried out. However, in several recent investigations (Diamond, 1972; Kinney, 1969; Sachs, 1969, 1971; Sachs & Anderson, 1967), attempts were made to teach subjects how to respond to other types of test suggestions. In several studies (Kinney, 1969; Sachs, 1971; Sachs & Anderson, 1967), the training procedures included the following: The experimenter described to the subject the sensations that he was expected to experience and he also utilized actual physical stimuli to help the subject understand what he was expected to experience. For instance, to acquaint the subject with the sensation of arm heaviness, heavy objects were piled on his hand. In addition, the subject was given verbal encouragement for successful responses and was allowed to practice each test suggestion at this own pace. Diamond (1972) used somewhat different procedures. For instance, he asked the subjects to listen to a responsive hypnotic subject who described how he thought and imagined when he passed the test suggestions. Similarly, in the proposed course that we outlined in Chapter 10 of this text, the experimenter explains to the subjects why learning to respond to suggestions is useful in fulfilling their potentialities and then he himself shows the subjects how they can respond to self-administered suggestions by thinking and imagining in certain ways. The investigations by Diamond (1972), Kinney (1969), and Sachs (1971), which included an evaluation of the effectiveness of the procedures, showed that the training was generally effective in enhancing the subjects' ability to pass test suggestions. Diamond (1972) found that the best results were obtained when the subjects who served as models not only performed the overt behaviors that were suggested but also reported in detail what they were thinking or imagining while they were responding to the suggestion. For instance, the model would describe how he passed a test suggestion to hallucinate music by stating: "[I] let myself imagine some music playing, like Dylan's *Mr. Tambourine Man*. I don't worry whether or not the music is coming from 'inside me' or from the outside, but just hear it as it is."

From our theoretical perspective, the training procedures used in the above investigations can be viewed as techniques for producing positive attitudes, motivations, and expectancies (cf. Kinney, 1969, pp. 38-41) and for teaching the subjects how to devise and implement cognitive strategies for passing test suggestions. The success of these procedures seems to lend support to our hypothesis that the cognitive strategies used by responsive subjects in hypnotic experiments can be taught to subjects who are initially unresponsive.[2]

Although we have used selective amnesia for a specific number to illustrate how cognitive strategies might be investigated, it should be clear that the same type of research procedures can also be used to investigate how subjects think and imagine when they pass other types of test suggestions. For instance, a systematic research program aimed at determining the kinds of cognitive strategies used by subjects to tolerate pain-producing stimulation should prove useful. As discussed in Chapter 10 of this text, our research indicates that subjects who are responsive to suggestions for anesthesia or analgesia commonly carry out one or more of the following cognitive strategies: they think of other things during the pain stimulation, or they imagine that the stimulated body part is made of rubber or is a lump of insensitive matter or has been injected with Novocain or, in some other way, has become numb and insensitive. Further research that checks and extends these findings should prove valuable not only for understanding hypnotism but also for providing useful methods for controlling pain.

As we noted previously, the presence or absence of an explicit cognitive strategy is not the only factor that determines whether or not test suggestions are difficult to experience. Another aspect of test suggestions that appears to be related to their level of difficulty is the extent to which they require the subject to ignore or reinterpret information that contradicts the effect that is being suggested. Let us look at this aspect in more detail.

Information Contradicting the Suggested Effect

When a subject is responding to test suggestions, he may be exposed to information that contradicts the very effect that the suggestion is attempting to engender. For example, let us suppose that a subject holds his arm outstretched and is then asked to imagine that a balloon is tied to the wrist and is making his arm light. Since the subject's arm is being held outstretched, it will be pulled downward by gravity. The subject will receive sensations from his arm indicating that it is feeling heavier rather than lighter. In other words, the subject will receive feedback from the muscles of his arm that is inconsistent with the suggestion that the arm is weightless and is being pulled upward by a balloon. In order to experience the arm as light and as rising involuntarily in the air, the subject must somehow ignore or reinterpret the incoming information that indicates his arm is actually feeling heavier and is tending to move downward. Suggestions differ in the extent to which they expose the subject to inconsistent or contradictory information. We can hypothesize that those test suggestions that expose the subject to the most inconsistent information are also the most difficult to pass. Let us look at some examples.

Weitzenhoffer and Hilgard (1962) have provided information concerning the proportion of hypnotic subjects who pass each of the test suggestions included in the Stanford Hypnotic Susceptibility Scale—Form C. The test suggestion for arm lowering asks the subject to imagine that he is holding a heavy weight in his outstretched hand and the weight is making the arm heavy and is bringing it down. An overwhelming majority of the subjects (92%) passed this test suggestion. The test suggestion for arm rigidity asks the subject to imagine that his arm is in a cast that prevents the elbow from bending. Only 45% of the subjects passed this test suggestion.

Why is the suggestion for arm lowering very easy to pass while the suggestion for arm rigidity is more difficult? Certainly it is not because the overt behaviors required by the two types of suggestions vary in difficulty to any significant degree—an individual can as easily lower his arm as he can make his arm rigid. Nor can we look to the presence or absence of cognitive strategies implied or stated in the suggestions to account for their different levels of difficulty. Each of the test suggestions asks the subject to carry out goal-directed imagining that can be helpful in experiencing the effects that are suggested; specifically, the suggestion for arm lowering asks the subject to imagine a heavy weight that is lowering his arm and the suggestion for arm rigidity asks the subject to imagine a cast that is keeping his arm rigid. Although both of these suggestions explicitly provide the subject with a cognitive strategy, they differ in the extent to which their enactment exposes the subject to information that is inconsistent with the suggested effect. Let us examine each of these test suggestions in more detail.

When exposed to the suggestion for arm lowering, the subject sits quietly with his arm outstretched and his eyes closed. As the force of gravity begins making his outstretched arm feel heavier, he is asked to imagine a weight pressing down on his arm. Thus, his imaginings are not contradicted by the sensory information from his arm. On the contrary, his imaginings and the sensory information are harmonious and reinforce one another.

In contrast, the suggestion for arm rigidity exposes the subject to contradictory information. When given the suggestion for arm rigidity, the subject is first asked to imagine a cast on his arm that keeps the elbow from bending and is then asked to try to bend the arm. In trying to bend the arm, the subject receives sensory information that contradicts the notion that his arm is held rigidly in a cast. He is exposed to feedback information indicating that there is no cast, no external object, that prevents his elbow from bending. Thus, in order to pass this test suggestion, the subject must ignore or reinterpret the sensory information that contradicts the idea of a cast holding the arm rigid.

In summary, these two test suggestions differ from one another in the extent to which their enactment exposes the subject to sensory information that contradicts the experience that is being suggested. The test suggestion that exposes the subject to harmonious feedback is easy to pass and the one that exposes him to contradictory feedback is more difficult.

Interrelations Between Cognitive Strategies, Contradictory Information, and Initial Level of Responsiveness

We have proposed that at least two variables affect the level of difficulty of test suggestions: the extent to which the suggestions direct the subject to employ a cognitive strategy and the degree to which they expose the subject to contradictory information. As yet, there are no systematically gathered data concerning the way these variables are interrelated. The collection of such data should prove fruitful. For instance, useful data can be provided by studies designed to test the hypothesis that an explicitly-stated cognitive strategy is more important in helping subjects to experience the suggested effect when the test suggestion exposes the subject to much rather than little contradictory information.

The two factors discussed above—presence of cognitive strategy and level of contradictory information—may exert different effects on subjects who are and those who are not initially responsive to test suggestions. For example, highly responsive subjects may find it easy to improvise their own cognitive strategies and, consequently, may gain little benefit from a cognitive strategy that is provided by the suggestion. On the other hand, subjects who manifest a low level of responsiveness to suggestions may find it difficult to improvise their own cognitive strategies and, consequently, may benefit from a cognitive strategy that is contained in the suggestion. It might prove fruitful to investigate this hypothesized interrelationship between subjects' initial level of suggestibility, presence of a cognitive strategy, and level of contradictory information.

Ignoring or Reinterpreting Contradictory Information

In the above discussion, we emphasized that the level of contradictory information to which a suggestion exposes the subject is one of the variables affecting its level of difficulty. Looked at from another angle, it appears likely that subjects who pass difficult test suggestions can more easily ignore or reinterpret contradictory information than those who fail difficult suggestions.

In Chapter 7, we summarized a recent experiment (Spanos, Ham, & Barber, 1973) that provided some data pertaining to the process of ignoring or reinterpreting contradictory information. The reader will recall that the subjects in this experiment were first given a very difficult suggestion for visual hallucination (to look at their lap for 30 seconds and see a cat sitting there) under a control (base-line) condition. Next, the subjects were exposed either to task motivational instructions or to a hypnotic induction procedure and then were given an equally difficult suggestion for visual hallucination (to look at their lap for 30 seconds and see a puppy dog sitting there). These suggestions implicitly asked the subjects to do two things: (a) to imagine or visualize an object on his lap and (b) to ignore or reinterpret incoming visual information telling him that his lap is actually empty.

A small proportion of subjects stated, during the experiment, that they saw the (suggested) object and, in addition, believed, part of the time, that it was actually "out there." These kinds of reports were given by 1% of the subjects under the control (base-line) condition, 3% under the task motivational condition, and 5% under the hypnotic induction condition. An interesting finding here is that the subjects who reported that they *saw* the (suggested) object and *believed* "part of the time" that it was "out there," described the (suggested) object in the same way as subjects who simply said that they *vividly imagined* it. Both sets of subjects described it as equally vague, transparent, weightless, unstable, etc. However, the subjects who reported that they saw it and believed "part of the time" that it was "out there" apparently ignored or reinterpreted the contradictory information. During postexperimental interviews, these subjects indicated that, when they were given the suggestion to see the object, they concentrated on imagining it and, while doing so, were not concerned with whether or not what they were imagining was "real"' Apparently, these subjects were able to ignore or reinterpret the contradictory information in somewhat the same way as a person who is reading an interesting novel or is observing an interesting motion picture is able to ignore or reinterpret contradictory information and not say to himself, "These are only symbols on a printed page," "These are only lights on a screen," "This is only a story that someone made up," or "These are only actors playing a part."

How can we obtain a broader understanding of the processes involved in ignoring or reinterpreting contradictory information while one is responding to suggestions; We agree with J.R. Hilgard (1970), Shor (1970), and other investigators that deeper insight into these processes can be gained by studying similar processes that occur when a person is engaged in other types of activities that also involve imagining. Let us briefly summarize some of the pertinent data.

The Relationship Between Responsiveness to Suggestions and Involvement in Imaginative Activities

A series of earlier studies (Andersen, 1963; As, 1962; As, O'Hara, & Munger, 1962; Barber & Glass, 1962: Coe, 1964; Lee-Teng, 1965; Shor, Orne, & O'Connell, 1962) and several recent studies (Atkinson, 1971; J.R. Hilgard, 1970; Spanos & McPeake, 1973b; Tellegen & Atkinson, 1972) indicate that individuals who are responsive to difficult test suggestions differ from those who are unresponsive in that they tend to become involved in activities that include imagining together with a "willing suspension of disbelief." For instance, Barber and Glass (1962) found that "highly suggestible" subjects gave more Yes answers than "unsuggestible" subjects to the following questionnaire items: "You like to read true stories about love and romance," "You find daydreaming very enjoyable," and "When you were a child of about five or six, did you have imaginary playmates who were rather vivid and almost real?" Along similar lines, both Andersen (1963) and Coe (1964) found that items such as the following are related to responsiveness to suggestions: "I find pure fantasy more enjoyable than fantasy utilizing realism to give it structure" and "I would like to get beyond the world of logic and reason and experience something different."

J.R. Hilgard (1970) has amplified the data, indicating that individuals who are responsive to suggestions in a hypnotic situation differ from those who are unresponsive in that they tend to become involved in activities that are based on imagining. Such "imaginative activities" include reading a novel, acting in a play, or listening to music. For example, one of J.R. Hilgard's responsive hypnotic subjects reported the following experience after reading Orwell's *1984*.

I identify myself with the character in *1984*, with Winston Smith, who was tortured at the end, fearing rats. His head was in a cage and he felt he would have to submit. I *felt* the fear that he felt as it came closer, closer. Walking back from the Union after finishing the book I had a problem relating myself to my present environment, to the stuff around me, for I was so entangled in the story that I had become exhausted [p.26].

Reports such as these, which pertain to involvement in imaginative activities such as reading a novel or acting in a drama, seem to resemble the statements made by subjects when they pass difficult test suggestions. In both cases, the subjects indicate that they were "carried away" by imaginings that were triggered by an outside source and, while doing so, were not concerned about the "reality" of their imaginings. Along similar lines, a series of studies (E.R. Hilgard, 1965; J.R. Hilgard, 1970; J.R. Hilgard & E.R. Hilgard, 1962) indicated that responsive hypnotic subjects tended to have experiences such as the following when they were children: they had imaginary companions and they were encouraged by their parents to become involved in listening to fairy tales.

J.R. Hilgard (1970) also found that unresponsive hypnotic subjects typically do not become involved in imaginative activities such as reading, dramatic acting, or listening to music. Instead, when engaged in such activities, they seem to keep their imaginings in check and do not allow themselves to be "carried off" by their imaginings.

In brief, there appears to be a relationship between responsiveness to test suggestions in a hypnotic situation and propensity for involvement in imaginative activities such as reading, dramatic acting, and listening to music. However, the relationship that seems to exist between these variables can be easily obscured or minimized by another set of variables. Let us explain.

An individual may have a propensity to become involved in various imaginative activities and yet may respond very poorly to test suggestions in a hypnotic situation. Why? As we have previously emphasized, such an individual may be unresponsive to test suggestions because of negative attitudes, motivations, or expectancies toward "hypnosis." For example, let us suppose that an individual who has a propensity to become involved in reading, dramatic acting, and other imaginative activities also prides himself on his spontaneity and independence. Let us further assume that this individual views "hypnosis" as a situation in which one person controls another's mind and in which the subject is forced against his will to act like a helpless automaton. Even though this individual is able to become involved in various imaginative activities, his negative attitudes toward "hypnosis" will most likely prevent him from responding to the test suggestions.

The above conjecture was recently tested experimentally. Working with 86 students, Spanos and McPeake (1973a) first administered a questionnaire that assessed propensity to become involved in everyday imaginative activities. Next, half of the subjects were given information intended to produce positive attitudes toward hypnosis; these subjects were told that hypnosis is interesting and useful, is not mysterious or dangerous, etc. The other half of the subjects were given negative information emphasizing that hypnotic responsiveness is a sign of gullibility and weakmindedness. All subjects were then tested for hypnotic suggestibility. Propensity to become involved in everyday imaginative activities was significantly correlated with hypnotic suggestibility ($r = .41$) in those subjects who had been given favorable information that would lead them to adopt positive attitudes toward hypnosis. However, propensity to become involved in imaginative activities was unrelated to hypnotic suggestibility ($r = .17$) when an attempt was made to induce negative attitudes toward hypnosis. The study also indicated that some subjects with a strong propensity for becoming involved in imaginative activities exhibit little hypnotic suggestibility because they hold negative attitudes toward the hypnotic situation.

The relationship between responsiveness to test suggestions in a hypnotic situation and ability to become involved in imaginative activities can also be tested by another kind of research strategy. This study would utilize subjects who are low in responsiveness to test suggestions and low in propensity for involvement in imaginative activities. Half of the subjects would be exposed to training procedures aimed at enhancing their ability to become involved in one of the imaginative activities—for example, in dramatic acting. These subjects could watch and listen to role models who are high in dramatic acting ability describe their experiences after playing a scene. The role models could describe their identification with the characters they are playing, the emotions they experienced, the means by which they tried to get "inside" the character, and their methods for ignoring or reinterpreting information that contradicted their role performance. The subjects could then play the same role while attempting to develop and maintain a perspective similar to that of the role models. The other half of the subjects, used as controls, would spend an equivalent amount of time in some unrelated activity. Both groups would then be retested to determine to what extent responsiveness to test suggestions is enhanced by training in the imaginative activity of dramatic acting.[3]

RELATING HYPNOTISM TO OTHER AREAS OF PSYCHOLOGY

A conspicuous characteristic of research in the area of hypnotism is its relative isolation from empirical and theoretical work in other areas of psychology. The reason for this is not too difficult to discern. Until quite recently, research in hypnotism has been dominated by the notion of a special state that gives rise to extraordinary experiences and behaviors. For over a century, this "hypnotic trance" point of view became so ingrained and commonplace that it was almost unthinkingly taken for granted as the "obvious" explanation of the phenomena associated with hypnotism. From this taken-for-granted "hypnotic trance" perspective, "hypnotic" phenomena could not be readily integrated into general psychology because these phenomena were thought to differ fundamentally from those studied by psychologists interested in such traditional topics as learning, perception, cognition, attitude change, social learning, psychotherapy, and the like.

The cognitive-behavioral viewpoint we have adopted suggests that "hypnotic" phenomena can be understood in terms of the same kinds of antecedent and mediating variables that are used to explain many other psychological phenomena. In other words, this point of view stresses that "hypnotic" phenomena and many other phenomena studied by psychologists may share a number of commonalities. The elucidation of such commonalities may help us develop a more general theory of psychology.

An Example: Relating Hypnotism to a Specific Therapeutic Procedure (Systematic Desensitization)

To illustrate how our viewpoint might clarify other areas of psychology, we shall compare the mediating variables involved in hypnotic situations with those involved in the therapeutic situation that has been labeled *systematic desensitization*. By disregarding the misleading notion of "hypnotic trance," we believe that commonalities in these two situations can come to light that would otherwise be obscured. Before discussing the variables that are common to these situations, we shall briefly familiarize the reader with the therapeutic procedures that are used in systematic desensitization.

Systematic desensitization is a treatment procedure that has been found to be especially useful in helping patients overcome their fears and phobias (Franks, 1969; Wolpe, 1958, 1969). The procedure usually involves three steps. First, the patient's fears are organized along a hierarchy starting with those fearful situations that produce only slight anxiety and going to those situations that produce a high degree of fear or panic. For example, if a patient has a fear of riding in airplanes, the first (least frightening) situation listed on his hierarchy might involve his approaching a sign that reads *Airport*. The last (most frightening) situation on the hierarchy might be the patient sitting in a plane that is traveling several thousand feet in the air. Between these extremes might be situations such as watching a plane take off, boarding a plane, and the like.

Once a fear hierarchy is constructed, the second step in the systematic desensitization procedure is to teach the patient how to achieve a high degree of relaxation. Finally, while remaining relaxed, the patient is asked to imagine each situation on the hierarchy beginning with the situation that created the least anxiety and going through to the situation that created the most anxiety. Patients who complete the desensitization sequence—that is, patients who are finally able to imagine the most frightening situation on the hierarchy while remaining relaxed—often overcome their fears.

In order to understand the behavior change found in systematic desensitization, we believe that the following three sets of variables that are present in desensitization situations (and also in hypnotic situations) should be taken into account: (a) subjects' attitudes, motivations, and expectancies toward the situation, (b) the specific wording of the suggestions or instructions that are administered, and (c) the extent to which the subject thinks and imagines with the themes that are suggested (Spanos, DeMoor, & Barber, 1973). Much of the present volume has been devoted to showing how these variables relate to performance in a hypnotic situation. Let us now look at the evidence indicating their importance in the desensitization situation.

Attitudes, motivations, and expectancies. A series of clinical reports and experimental studies indicate that these variables are important in determining how much therapeutic improvement is shown by patients when they undergo systematic desensitization. Thus, therapists using desensitization often provide patients with instructions aimed at enhancing their attitudes and motivations (Brown, 1967; Klein, Dittman, Parloff, & Gill, 1969; Wolpe, 1958); a number of therapists have attested to the fact that desensitization is of little benefit when patients have negative attitudes or motivations toward it. For instance, Lazarus (1971) indicated that desensitization is only effective with patients "who do not derive too much primary or secondary gains from their avoidance behavior" and "who are not strongly averse to the method" (p. 95).

Recently, a series of experiments (e.g., Leitenberg, Agras, Barlow, & Oliveau, 1969; Miller, 1972; Oliveau, Agras, Leitenberg, Moore, & Wright, 1969) indicated the importance of the patients' expectancies in affecting the outcome of desensitization. In these experiments, patients in one group were told that they would undergo therapy that would help them overcome their fear of snakes. These patients then underwent desensitization. The other group of patients also underwent desensitization, but they were not told that they were undergoing therapy for their fears. Instead, the desensitization procedure was explained to the latter group as being part of an experiment dealing with imagination and physiological responsiveness. The desensitization procedure was markedly more effective in reducing fear of snakes when the patients expected that the procedure would help them overcome their fears. These experiments indicate that in the desensitization situation, as in the hypnotic situation, subjects' expectations play an important role in determining how they will respond.

Wording of suggestions or instructions. In earlier chapters, we indicated that the experiences and behaviors that occurred in hypnotic situations were related to the wording of the suggestions that the subjects were given. The same variable also seems to play a role in the desensitization situation (Spanos, DeMoor, & Barber, 1973). The specific instructions used in desensitization, like the suggestions used in the hypnotic situation, usually do not ask the patient to carry out an overt behavior. Instead, they ask the patient to imagine vividly a set of hypothetical events and they imply that these imaginings will produce changes in behavior. For example, a patient undergoing desensitization for a snake phobia is never told, "You are not afraid of snakes. Go up and touch the snake." Instead, he is told something like, "Imagine that you are standing at one end of a long corridor. At the other end of the corridor is a large, nonpoisonous black snake. Now, imagine yourself taking a step down the corridor toward the snake."

Thinking and vividly imagining with the themes of the suggestions or instructions. The insistence of behavior therapists that vivid and realistic imagery is a prerequisite for successful desensitization (Wolpe, 1958, 1969)[4] and the attempts of such therapists to get their patients to "really feel" the suggested effects (Cautela, 1971) indicate that involvement in imagining is also an important dimension in desensitization. Although more data are needed before any conclusions can be drawn, we would hypothesize that, other things being equal, patients who are more able to become involved in or to concentrate on their imaginings will fare better in desensitization.

Let us state one final commonality. We pointed out earlier that hypnotic subjects who successfully pass test suggestions sometimes imagine situations that differ from the situations that are suggested but that are goal-directed nevertheless in that, if the situation that was imagined were to actually occur, it would tend to give rise to the suggested behavior. Interestingly enough, the little evidence available (Barrett, 1969; Brown, 1967; Weinberg & Zaslove, 1963; Weitzman, 1967) indicates that patients undergoing systematic desensitization also often imagine situations that are goal-directed but quite different from the specific events that they are instructed to imagine. It remains to be determined whether this kind of goal-directed imagining plays an important role in producing the desired therapeutic change in desensitization.

Our purpose has not been to show that hypnotism and desensitization are "the same thing" or that the only variables that produce therapeutic change in desensitization are also found in hypnotic situations. Instead, we have tried to show that (a) these situations contain a number of commonalities that are important in understanding the behavior change seen in each situation, (b) these commonalities have not been fully appreciated because the "hypnotic trance" notion tends to preclude looking for these kinds of similarities between hypnotism and other research areas that deal with "normal" phenomena, and (c) a free flow of information between these research areas, unencumbered by the "hypnotic trance" notion, will lead to a mutual theoretical enhancement.

Another Illustrative Example: Relating Hypnotism to Social Psychology

As another example, let us look at how hypnotism can be related to social psychology. The mediating variables discussed in this text—attitudes, motivations, expectancies, and cognitive processes such as thinking and imagining—are an integral part of present-day social psychology. Also, the area subsumed under the term "hypnotism" is a social psychological phenomenon *par excellence* in that one individual exerts a potent influence on the behavior and experience of another individual. Consequently, it is rather surprising that recent texts in social psychology do not deal with hypnotism even though they usually deal in detail with such topics as persuasion, conformity, and attitude change. It appears that the area of hypnotism is typically viewed by social psychologists as falling outside of their domain—as falling more closely in the areas of abnormal psychology or psychiatry that cover "trances" and other "special states."

With one limited exception (McGuire, 1968), no attempt has been made by social psychologists to integrate under a unified framework such phenomena as persuasion, conformity, attitude change, and hypnotism or suggestibility. However, from our point of view, each of these social psychological phenomena involve overlapping processes; further efforts to tie them together conceptually should prove extremely fruitful.

Fortunately, one very useful attempt to relate hypnotism to one kind of theoretical model in social psychology—the role model—has been made by Sarbin. Let us look briefly at Sarbin's important formulation.

Sarbin's social psychological formulation. Sarbin's formulation has many points in common with the cognitive-behavioral formulation we have presented in this text. Sarbin and his associates (Sarbin, 1950a; Sarbin & Andersen, 1967; Sarbin & Coe, 1972) also view concepts such as *hypnotic trance* or *hypnotic state* as misleading in trying to explain the phenomena associated with hypnotism. In addition, they have tried to show that "hypnotic" phenomena are not unique or isolated from other kinds of social psychological phenomena.

Although there are many points in common between Sarbin's formulation and ours, they differ in that Sarbin's formulation pivots around the concept of *role*. Sarbin views the subject in a hypnotic situation as striving to take the role of a hypnotized person. He points out that in our culture everyone has a general conception of the role of a hypnotic subject—that is, how a hypnotized person is supposed to behave. In addition, the role is defined more specifically by the instructions and suggestions of the hypnotist. As an analogy, Sarbin refers to the actor who strives to take the role that is assigned to him. When an actor is able to become involved in his role, he may cry with real tears and may laugh, feel, emote, and experience the part he is playing. Also, when the actor becomes involved in his role, his concentration and attention may become focalized on a rather narrow range and he may tend to lose awareness of "self." Sarbin notes that when the subject in a hypnotic situation becomes involved in the role of the hypnotized person, he may, in a similar manner, show focalized attention and may tend to lose self-awareness or self-consciousness.

From Sarbin's viewpoint (Sarbin & Andersen, 1967), the subject's success in taking the role of the hypnotized person is dependent on such variables as the following: (a) his role expectations (how he expects to behave in the hypnotic situation), (b) his role perception (how he interprets the hypnotist's statements defining how he is to behave and what he is to experience), (c) his role-relevant skills (such as his ability to imagine vividly), (d) his self-role congruence (that is, whether his understanding of what is required of a hypnotic subject is discrepant from or in harmony with his conception of himself as a person who behaves in certain ways), and (e) his sensitivity to role-demands (for example, his sensitivity to the fact that he will embarrass the hypnotist if he does not respond to his suggestions).

Clearly, Sarbin's formulation and our formulation have many points in common. Further attempts to integrate the two formulations may enhance progress in this area.

SUMMARY

Limitations of the cognitive-behavioral formulation were pointed out and areas of research were suggested that can further enhance our understanding of hypnotism. Four questions were at the forefront of discussion:

1. *How can we clarify the role of the complex conglomerate of variables that comprise an induction procedure?* Needed research was outlined that would focus on each variable separately and also on the additivity of the variables taken in combination. It was also noted that faster progress would be made in this area if relaxation-sleep-hypnosis suggestions were conceptualized as another set of test suggestions rather than as special suggestions that give rise to a special state. Finally, research

was outlined that might further clarify the role of the hypnotist and the relationship between the subject and the hypnotist.

2. *How can we delineate experimentally the relevance of subjects' attitudes, motivations, and expectancies?* Research was outlined that might clarify the relative importance of each of these three mediating variables and how the three variables are interrelated.

3. *How can we proceed to gain a deeper understanding of the processes involved in thinking and imagining with the themes of the suggestions?* Research was outlined that could enhance our understanding of (a) how responsive subjects utilize cognitive strategies to pass difficult test suggestions, (b) how responsive subjects succeeded in ignoring or reinterpreting information that contradicts the suggested effects, and (c) how responsiveness to test suggestions is related to ability to become involved in reading novels, acting in a play, and other activities that seem to involve imagining and "a willing suspension of disbelief."

4. *How can the area of hypnotism be integrated with other areas of psychology?* Data were presented indicating that, when we lay aside the misleading notion of "hypnotic trance," we can find previously unseen commonalities between the variables that mediate responsiveness to suggestions and the variables that mediate other psychological phenomena. As illustrative examples, the processes involved in hypnotic situations were compared with those involved in one type of therapeutic situation (systematic desensitization) and with those involved in several social psychological situations. Also, while discussing the integration of hypnotism with social psychology, Sarbin's important social psychological formulation of hypnotism was summarized and was shown to have many commonalities with the cognitive-behavioral formulation presented in this text.

NOTES

[1] Responses to relaxation-sleep-hypnosis suggestions can be scored in several ways—for instance, by the subject's self-report, made immediately after he has received the suggestions, pertaining to the extent that he feels relaxed.

[2] Further studies are needed to delineate useful techniques for teaching individuals how to think and imagine in order to have the experiences that have been historically associated with the term "hypnotism." One way to proceed is to test the usefulness of the methods that were described in Chapter 10 in the course that we labeled *Training in Human Potentialities*. To what extent does the subject accept the definition of the situation as "training in human potentialities" and how does this way of defining the situation affect his attitudes, motivations, and expectancies? Also, is it more effective for the experimenter himself to serve as a model in showing the subject how to think and imagine in order to have the experiences or is it more useful for someone other than the experimenter to model for the subject?

[3] Of course, this research should also assess the subjects' attitudes, motivations, and expectancies toward "hypnosis" and toward responding to suggestions prior to and after the training in dramatic acting. This is necessary in order to determine whether any gain in responsiveness to suggestions is due to the training *per se* or to the training altering the subjects' attitudes, motivations, or expectancies toward responding to suggestions.

[4] Although "imagery" is involved in "imagining," these concepts are not synonymous. "Imagining" involves "visual imagery," but it also involves other complex cognitive processes that are analyzed by Juhasz (1969).

* * *

Hilgard extract is from Hilgard, J.R. *Personality and Hypnosis*. Chicago: University of Chicago Press, 1970.

Appendices

Appendix A

Barber Suggestibility Scale

The Barber Suggestibility Scale includes the following eight test suggestions:[1]

1. *Arm Lowering.* Starting with the subject's right arm extended and horizontal, suggestions are given for 30 seconds that the arm is becoming heavy and is moving down.

2. *Arm Levitation.* Starting with the subject's left arm horizontal, suggestions are given for 30 seconds that the arm is weightless and is moving up.

3. *Hand Lock.* The subject is instructed to clasp his hands together tightly with fingers intertwined and then suggestions are given for 45 seconds that the hands are welded together and cannot be taken apart.

4. *Thirst Hallucination.* The subject is told repeatedly for 45 seconds that he is becoming extremely thirsty.

5. *Verbal Inhibition.* Suggestions are given for 45 seconds that the subject's throat and jaw muscles are rigid and he cannot speak his name.

6. *Body Immobility.* Suggestions are given for 45 seconds that the subject's body is heavy and rigid and he cannot stand up.

7. *Posthypnotic-like Response.* The subject is told that, when the experiment is over, he will cough automatically when he hears a click.

8. *Selective Amnesia.* The subject is told that when the experiment is over, he will remember all of the test suggestions except the one instructing him to move his arm up (Arm Levitation), and then he will remember this test suggestion when he is given a cue word.

Responses to the test suggestions are scored in two ways—objectively and subjectively. With regard to *Objective* scores, the subject receives one point for

151

passing each test suggestion; thus, the subject can obtain a total Objective score on the Barber Suggestibility Scale ranging from 0 (passing none of the test suggestions) to 8 (passing all of them). The overt behaviors that are manifested when the subject passes each test suggestion objectively are as follows: his arm moved down four or more inches (Arm Lowering); his arm moved up four or more inches (Arm Levitation); he failed to unclasp his hands after 15 seconds of trying to do so (Hand Lock); he showed observable signs of thirst such as moistening of lips, marked mouth movements, or swallowing, and stated that he felt thirsty (Thirst Hallucination); he did not say his name even though he tried to say it for at least 15 seconds (Verbal Inhibition); he was not standing erect from the chair after 15 seconds of trying to stand erect (Body Immobility); he coughed or cleared his throat postexperimentally when presented with the click stimulus (Posthypnotic-like Response); and he did not refer to the item that was to be forgotten, but mentioned at least four other items and then recalled the "forgotten" item when given the cue word (Selective Amnesia).

The Barber Suggestibility Scale also contains provisions for assessing *Subjective* responses to the test suggestions. After the subjects are tested for overt response to the test suggestions, they are asked whether they actually experienced each suggested effect or if they went along with the suggestion in order to follow instructions or to please the experimenter. A Subjective score of 1 point is assigned for each of the eight test suggestions that the subject states he actually experienced. Thus, the subject can obtain a total Subjective score on the Barber Suggestibility Scale ranging from 0 (experiencing none of the suggested effects) to 8 (experiencing all of them).[2]

NOTES

[1] A complete word-by-word account of the Barber Suggestibility Scale is presented by Barber (1965a, 1969b) and Barber and Calverley (1963a).

[2] More recently, another method has been developed for scoring subjective responses to the Barber Suggestibility Scale (Barber and Calverley, 1966c, p. 423).

Appendix B

Surgery with Acupuncture

In Chapter 8 we explained how the pain of surgery is attenuated in situations that involve hypnotism and suggestions. The factors delineated in Chapter 8 also help explain how surgical pain is relieved by acupuncture. Before summarizing the explanation of "acupuncture anesthesia," which we have presented in detail elsewhere (Barber, 1973a; Chaves, 1972; Chaves & Barber, 1973), let us briefly describe acupuncture.

ACUPUNCTURE

Acupuncture is an ancient Chinese method of therapy that involves the insertion of thin needles into precise points on the body. It appears that the technique of acupuncture has existed in China for at least 5000 years. It was originally used for treatment of specific illnesses such as arthritic disorders and gastrointestinal diseases (Veith, 1972). During very recent years (since 1959), it has also been used as an anesthetic in surgery.

An elaborate theory determines where on the body the needles are to be placed. This theory, which is described in detail by Drake (1972) and Mann (1962), is based on the concepts of *Yin* and *Yang*. Yin is the weak, female, negative force; Yang is the strong, male, positive force. Health is viewed as a condition of harmony between Yin and Yang, while disease is thought to result from an imbalance of these two forces. Yin and Yang control life energy *(Ch'i)*, which flows from organ to organ in the body through a network of meridians or channels *(Ching-lo)* that lie beneath the skin. During treatment, acupuncture needles are placed along the meridians at points that are thought to correspond to specific organs. However, these points are not located at the same anatomical sites as the organs they are supposed to affect; for instance, both rectal hemorrhoids and blurred vision may be treated by placing an acupuncture needle in the leg.

Recent writers have criticized the ancient Chinese theory that determines where the needles are inserted. Mann (1972), who has closely studied the topic and who has written many books about it, has recently stated that "... I don't believe meridians exist. A lot of acupuncture is based on meridians, and you will see from my theory, I think the meridians of acupuncture are not very much more real than the meridians of geography. And likewise with the acupuncture points" (p. 30). Mann (1972) has also noted that "The Chinese have so many interconnections in their acupuncture theory that one can explain everything just as politicians do" (p. 24). Somewhat more succinctly, Wall (1972) has stated, with regard to the meridians: "There is not one scrap of anatomical or physiological evidence for the existence of such a system" (p. 129). Along similar lines, Man and Chen (1972) have pointed out that some Chinese surgeons "totally disregarded the recognized spots on the meridians" and used almost any spot to produce "surgical anesthesia."

Although the theory that underlies acupuncture may be invalid, the acupuncture technique itself seems to have useful effects. When acupuncture is used to attenuate pain during surgery, the technique for needle placement involves the following: The acupuncture needles are rarely if ever inserted near vital organs, and they are rarely inserted more than an inch below the skin. The needles are inserted at points that are distant from the surgical site; for example, when abdominal surgery is performed, the needles may be placed in the ear, the arm, or the head (Tkach, 1972). In recent years, it has become common practice to apply electric current to the needles or to twirl and vibrate them by hand. The needles are continuously manipulated for at least 20 minutes and "the patient must feel sore, distended, heavy, and numb over the site of needle placement" (Chen, 1972, p. 81).

As stated previously, the use of acupuncture in surgery is rather recent. Hendin (1972) has pointed out that in China "acupuncture has been used as an anesthetic only since 1959." Although the use of acupuncture in surgery is a new development, it has recently received more attention in medical journals than has its ancient use to treat specific diseases (Freedman, 1972; Kroger, 1972a, 1972b; Liu, 1972; Matsumoto, 1972; Wolffenbüttel, 1968). We believe that our explanation of "suggested or hypnotic anesthesia," presented in Chapter 8, may also be useful in explaining "acupuncture anesthesia." We shall now attempt to explain the attenuation of surgical pain that is associated with acupuncture in much the same way that we explained the reduction of surgical pain that is associated with hypnotism and suggestions. First, we shall discuss four points that are relevant to understanding the effects of acupuncture in surgery: (a) patients are selected who are low in anxiety and who have positive attitudes, motivations, and expectancies toward the acupuncture situation; (b) the patients are exposed to pre-operative training and preparation; (c) pain-relieving drugs are used along with the acupuncture; and (d) failures occur during acupuncture surgery. After we have amplified these four points, we shall discuss the effects of (e) distraction and (f) suggestions and, finally, we shall look once again at (g) the base-level of surgical pain.

PATIENT SELECTION: LOW ANXIETY AND POSITIVE ATTITUDES, MOTIVATIONS, AND EXPECTANCIES

Recent newspaper reports imply that acupuncture is routinely employed in China with surgical patients. This impression is false. Dimond (1971) has pointed out that "The decision to use acupuncture anesthesia depended on the full enthusiasm and acceptance by the patient." Patients who are frightened and tense are given general anesthesia. Warren (1972) has noted that surgeons select patients for acupuncture according to the following criteria: "They decide whether the type of operation would be suitable, whether the patient would be too hysterical, whether the patient believes firmly in Mao's teaching, or would Mao's teaching carry him through" (p. 88).

It should be emphasized that patients appear to be motivated to undergo surgery with acupuncture because of the "immense pressure to comply and participate in the current Mao Thought program which is a fundamental requirement for life in China" (Dimond, 1971, p. 1560). As Kroger (1972b) has pointed out, "Specific factors responsible for acupuncture anesthesia are: the antecedent variables such as the generalized stoicism of the Chinese, the ideological zeal, the evangelical fervor, the prior beliefs shared by *acupuncteurists* and patients. . . . *Mao Tse-tung's New Thought Directives* [and the] ceremonial-like placement of the needles . . ." (p. 3). The patients who are selected to undergo surgery with acupuncture while being observed by Western physicians may be especially motivated to do well. At the completion of the surgery, the patients observed by Dimond (1971) and Tkach (1972) thanked Chairman Mao and some made statements such as "Long live Chairman Mao and welcome American doctors."

Although precise data on the numbers and kinds of patients who undergo surgery with acupuncture are not available, it seems clear that the patients are carefully selected. Patients who are anxious or who have negative attitudes, motivations, or expectancies do not undergo surgery with acupuncture; instead, they are given general anesthesia. We have seen from our discussion in Chapter 8 that low levels of anxiety and positive attitudes, motivations, and expectancies are generally associated with a reduction in pain.

PREOPERATIVE PREPARATION

The selected patient typically comes to the hospital two days before the surgery and the surgeons explain to him exactly what they are going to do, show him how they will operate, and explain to him what the acupuncturist will do and what effects the needles will have (Tkach, 1972). The patient is asked to talk to other patients who have had the same kind of surgery and he is also given a set of acupuncture needles so that he can try them on himself (Tkach, 1972). This preoperative preparation of the patient appears to be a useful method for reducing anxiety and fear (Egbert, Battit, Turndorf, & Beecher, 1963; Egbert, Battit, Welch, & Bartlett, 1964). Also, prior to surgery, the patients are typically given training on how to control their breathing (Warren, 1972). By focusing their attention on their breathing during the surgery, the patients may be distracted from the effects of the surgeon's incisions.

USE OF PAIN-RELIEVING DRUGS

Recent newspaper reports imply that, when acupuncture is used in surgery, pain-relieving drugs are not employed. A careful examination of individual case reports indicates that this implication is false. Of the six cases reported by Dimond (1971), for example, three received 50-60 mg. of meperidine hydrochloride (Demerol) by intravenous drip, one received 10 mg. of morphine, and another patient who had received 0.3 mg. of scopolamine was also given an injection of procaine (Novocain) into the peritoneal cavity when he complained of pain. Not only is Demerol commonly administered in an intravenous drip in doses of 50 or 60 mg. (Man & Chen, 1972), but morphine (10 mg.) is also at times injected at acupuncture points.

When acupuncture is employed for brain operations, surgeons typically infiltrate the scalp with procaine before the incision is made (Brown, 1972; Capperauld, 1972). Capperauld (1972) noted that acupuncture patients generally receive sedative doses of barbiturates prior to surgery and intravenous meperidine hydrochloride (Demerol) and promethazine hydrochloride during surgery. Capperauld also observed that local anesthetics were frequently used to dull the pain of the initial incision through the skin. Since narcotic analgesics, sedatives, and local anesthetics are commonly administered to patients undergoing surgery with acupuncture, it is very difficult to determine whether any additional pain relief is contributed by the acupuncture needles themselves

FAILURES WITH ACUPUNCTURE

Although the success of acupuncture in producing anesthesia during surgery has gone virtually unchallenged in the popular press, available case reports indicate that failures occur. For instance, Dimond (1971) reported that one of six selected patients complained of pain, and he stated that acupuncture also failed to relieve pain in other surgical patients; that is, the patients experienced intolerable pain or were too tense and additional pain-relieving drugs had to be administered. In the remaining cases, it appeared that acupuncture together with some pain-relieving drug, such as 50 mg. of Demerol administered intravenously, was sufficient for the patients to tolerate the surgery.

A recent experimental study indicates that acupuncture *per se* does not remove sensitivity to pain. The investigator (Mann, 1973), who is one of the foremost Western authorities on techniques of acupuncture, worked with 100 volunteer subjects in England. He tested the effectiveness of acupuncture in relieving the pain produced by repeated pinpricks on the skin that were severe enough to draw blood. Of the 100 subjects who were undergoing "acupuncture analgesia," 90 reported that the pinpricks hurt. Although the remaining 10 subjects did not report pain during "acupuncture analgesia," this does not necessarily mean that acupuncture is effective in removing pain in 10% of the population. As all pain researchers know, a certain percentage of the normal population (possibly as high as 10%) does not report pain when exposed to such noxious stimuli as pinpricks. Mann attributed the failure of acupuncture to the fact that, unlike the Chinese, he made no special effort to convince his subjects of the effectiveness of acupuncture in reducing pain.

DISTRACTION AND SUGGESTIONS

In addition to the factors discussed above, we need to consider two additional factors that appear to play an important role—distraction and suggestions.

Distraction. Although acupuncture needles are usually inserted at innocuous locations, their insertion and accompanying manual or electrical stimulation give rise to various sensations. At times, the electric current that is applied to the acupuncture needles is strong enough to produce rather strong muscle contractions (Tkach, 1972). Also, the needles are commonly manipulated for at least 20 minutes before surgery and they give rise to boring or aching sensations (Chen, 1972; Man & Chen, 1972). McGarey (1972) noted that "A deep but minimal aching sensation is often felt when the needle is properly placed" (p. 19). Furthermore, some patients report pain from the acupuncture needles. For instance, in describing his own experience with acupuncture for the relief of postoperative pain, Reston (1972) noted that the needles "sent ripples of pain racing through my limbs and, at least, had the effect of diverting my attention from the distress in my stomach." It appears that acupuncture needles can serve as distractors. It may be that they function as especially effective distractors when an electric current is applied to them. Evidence reviewed in Chapter 8 showed that distraction can be a potent variable in reducing reported pain.

Suggestions. It is clear that surgical patients who are accepted for acupuncture believe that acupuncture is effective in relieving pain. Furthermore, suggestions for pain relief are an integral part of the acupuncture situation. Even when acupuncture is used to treat specific diseases, Rhee (1972) observed that ". . . . the acupuncturists whom I have watched work, load their therapy with suggestions" (p. 10). A series of experimental studies that we reviewed in Chapter 8 indicated that suggestions for pain relief can be effective in reducing reported pain.

BASE-LEVEL OF SURGICAL PAIN

As was pointed out in Chapter 8, it appears that the pain of major surgery is less than is usually assumed. Major surgery can often be accomplished with pain that can be tolerated if local anesthetics such as Novocain are used to dull the pain of the initial incision. Furthermore, when patients are relaxed, it is often possible for them to tolerate major surgery with small doses of pain-relieving drugs or, in a small number of cases, with no drugs at all. Thus, it is unclear what the base-level of pain would be for patients undergoing the same types of surgery that are attempted with acupuncture, but without having the acupuncture needles inserted.[1]

It should be emphasized that although internal tissues and organs are largely insensitive to incision, they are sensitive to traction. When internal organs are stimulated by traction during surgery with acupuncture, the patients grimace, sweat, and show other signs of experiencing extreme distress (Capperauld, 1972).

SUMMARY AND CONCLUSION

The acupuncture situation involves a host of important variables that are known to reduce pain; low levels of patient anxiety and very positive attitudes, motivations, and expectancies; preoperative preparation of patients; training in breathing exercises; the use of small or moderate doses of pain-relieving drugs; distraction; and suggestions. Further research is needed to determine the relative contribution of each of these factors. Such research may identify other factors that may also help to account for "acupuncture analgesia." However, at the present time, there is no evidence that acupuncture needles exert specific analgesic effects beyond those we have discussed.[2]

NOTES

[1] Recent reports in the popular press state that acupuncture has been used to perform surgery on animals such as rabbits, cats, and mules. These anecdotal reports cannot be evaluated until such time as base-level reactions to pain are established in animals undergoing the same kinds of surgery without acupuncture needles. Since many mammals, including rabbits and horses, can tolerate extremely painful stimuli under certain conditions (Ratner, 1967), controlled studies may find that acupuncture per se is not particularly helpful in surgery with animals.

[2] Attempts to provide a scientific account of acupuncture frequently lead to a discussion of the Gate Control theory of pain proposed by Melzack and Wall (1965). Briefly, this theory asserts that pain depends in part on the relative balance of activity of large fibers, activated by nonpainful tactile stimuli, and small fibers, activated by pain-producing stimuli. Increasing activity of the large fibers is thought to close a "gate" in a part of the spinal column (the substantia gelatinosa) preventing the further transmission of information from the small "pain fibers." As applied to acupuncture, it is assumed that the needles selectively stimulate the large fibers and, thus, inhibit pain.

There are difficulties in using the Gate Control Theory to account for acupuncture anesthesia. First, in order to account for the efficacy of acupuncture needles inserted into the head or ears, it has been necessary to postulate the existence of a second "gate" located in the thalamus. This assumption is necessary since acupuncture needles in the head or ears would presumably be ineffective in closing the spinal "gate." Secondly, as Shealy (1972) and Wall (1972) have pointed out, the Gate Control theory can only account for local analgesia in the vicinity of the nerves stimulated by the acupuncture needles. However, acupuncture needles are typically placed in locations that are quite remote from the location where analgesia is desired. Wall (1972), the original coauthor of the Gate Control theory, has stated: "My present guess is that . . . it will emerge that acupuncture does not generate the specifically pain inhibiting barrages for which I was looking" (p. 130).

However, the other coauthor of the Gate Control theory has argued that the theory is relevant to acupuncture analgesia (Melzack, 1973). Perhaps the greatest challenge to the Gate Control theory is its inability to account for the failures with acupuncture. Why is it necessary for acupuncture patients to believe in its effectiveness (Mann, 1973)? If acupuncture produces analgesia by a direct physiological route, why is it necessary to screen patients so carefully? If acupuncture needles can really close the "gate" and thus inhibit pain, why is it necessary to use sedatives, narcotic analgesics, and local anesthetics in addition to the acupuncture needles? Why is the "gate" capable of reducing the pain of surgery in China, but incapable of reducing the pain of pinpricks in England (Mann, 1973)? The Gate Control theory fails to provide answers for these important questions. It appears to us that a search for a physiological explanation of "acupuncture analgesia" is premature.

References

Allington, H. V. Sulpharsphenamine in the treatment of warts. *Archives of Dermatology and Syphilology*, 1934, 29, 687-690.

Andersen, M. L. Correlates of hypnotic performance: An historical and role-theoretical analysis. Doctoral dissertation, University of California, 1963.

Anderson, M. N. Hypnosis in anesthesia. *Journal of the Medical Association of Alabama*, 1957, 27, 121-125.

Arnold, M. B. On the mechanisms of suggestion and hypnosis. *Journal of Abnormal and Social Psychology*, 1946, 41, 107-128.

Arons, H. *How to Routine an Ethical Hypnotic Lecture-Demonstration.* Irvington, N.J.: Power Publishers, 1961.

As, A. Non-hypnotic experiences related to hypnotizability in male and female college students. *Scandinavian Journal of Psychology*, 1962, 3, 112-121.

As, A., O'Hara, J.W., and Munger, M.P. The measurement of subjective experiences presumably related to hypnotic susceptibility. *Scandinavian Journal of Psychology*, 1962, 3, 47-64.

Ascher, L.M., Barber, T.X., and Spanos, N.P. Two attempts to replicate the Parrish-Lundy-Leibowitz experiment on hypnotic age regression. *American Journal of Clinical Hypnosis*, 1972, 14, 178-185.

Atkinson, G.A. Personality and hypnotic cognition. Doctoral dissertation, University of Minnesota, 1971.

August, R.V. *Hypnosis in Obstetrics.* New York: McGraw-Hill, 1961.

Balaschak, B., Blocker, K., Rossiter, T., and Perin, C.T. The influence of race and expressed experience of the hypnotist on hypnotic susceptibility. *International Journal of Clinical and Experimental Hypnosis*, 1972, 20, 38-45.

Barber, T.X. Hypnosis as perceptual-cognitive restructuring: II. "Post"-hypnotic behavior. *Journal of Clinical and Experimental Hypnosis*, 1958, 6, 10-20.

Barber, T.X. Toward a theory of pain: Relief of chronic pain by prefrontal leucotomy, opiates, placebos, and hypnosis. *Psychological Bulletin*, 1959, 56, 430-460.

Barber, T.X. Antisocial and criminal acts induced by "hypnosis": A review of clinical and experimental findings. *Archives of General Psychiatry*, 1961, 5, 301-312. (a)

Barber, T.X. Experimental evidence for a theory of hypnotic behavior: II. Experimental controls in hypnotic age-regression, *International Journal of Clinical and Experimental Hypnosis*, 1961, 9, 181-193 (b)

Barber, T.X. Physiological effects of "hypnosis." *Psychological Bulletin*, 1961, 58, 390-419. (c)

Barber, T.X. Hypnotic age regression: A critical review. *Psychosomatic Medicine*, 1962, 24, 286-299. (a)

Barber, T.X. Toward a theory of hypnosis: Posthypnotic behavior. *Archives of General Psychiatry*, 1962, 7, 321-342. (b)

Barber, T.X. The effect of "hypnosis" on pain: A critical review of experimental and clinical findings. *Psychosomatic Medicine*, 1963, 25, 303-333. [Reprinted in T.X. Barber et al. (Eds.) *Biofeedback and Self-Control: An Aldine Reader*. Chicago: Aldine-Atherton, 1971. Pp. 724-754.]

Barber, T.X. "Hypnosis" as a causal variable in present-day psychology: A critical analysis. *Psychological Reports*, 1964, 14, 839-842.

Barber, T.X. Measuring "hypnotic-like" suggestibility with and without "hypnotic induction"; psychometric properties, norms, and variables influencing response to the Barber Suggestibility Scale (BSS). *Psychological Reports*, 1965, 16, 809-844. (a)

Barber, T.X. Physiological effects of "hypnotic suggestions": A critical review of recent research (1960-64). *Psychological Bulletin*, 1965, 63, 201-222. (b)

Barber, T.X. Reply to Conn and Conn's "Discussion of Barber's 'hypnosis' as a causal variable . . ." *International Journal of Clinical and Experimental Hypnosis*, 1967, 15, 111-117.

Barber, T.X. Effects of hypnotic induction, suggestions of anesthesia, and distraction on subjective and physiological responses to pain. Paper presented at the annual meeting of the Eastern Psychological Association, Philadelphia, April 10, 1969. (a)

Barber, T.X. *Hypnosis: A Scientific Approach*. New York: Van Nostrand Reinhold, 1969. (b)

Barber, T.X. Review of "Advanced Techniques of Hypnosis and Therapy: Selected Papers by Milton H. Erickson, M.D." *Psychiatry*, 1969, 32, 221-225. (c)

Barber, T.X. *LSD, Marihuana, Yoga, and Hypnosis*. Chicago: Aldine, 1970.

Barber, T.X. Suggested ("hypnotic") behavior: The trance paradigm versus an alternative paradigm. In E. Fromm and R. E. Shor (Eds.) *Hypnosis: Research Developments and Perspectives*. Chicago: Aldine-Atherton, 1972. Pp. 115-182.

Barber, T.X. Acupuncture anesthesia in surgery: A scientific explanation. Paper presented at the Second Western Hemisphere Conference on Acupuncture, Kirlian Photography and the Human Aura, New York, February 13, 1973 (a)

Barber, T.X. Pitfalls in research: Nine investigator and experimenter effects. In R.M.W. Travers (Ed.) *Second Handbook of Research on Teaching*. Chicago: Rand McNally, 1973. Pp. 382-404. (b)

Barber, T.X., Ascher, L.M., and Mavroides, M. Effects of practice on hypnotic suggestibility: A re-evaluation of Hull's postulates. *American Journal of Clinical Hypnosis*, 1971, 14, 48-53.

Barber, T.X., and Calverley, D.S. "Hypnotic" behavior as a function of task motivation. *Journal of Psychology*, 1962, 54, 363-389.

Barber, T.X., and Calverley, D.S. "Hypnotic-like" suggestibility in children and adults. *Journal of Abnormal and Social Psychology*, 1963, 66, 589-597. (a)

Barber, T.X., and Calverley, D.S. The relative effectiveness of task motivating instructions and trance induction procedure in the production of "hypnotic-like" behaviors. *Journal of Nervous and Mental Disease*, 1963, 137, 107-116. (b)

Barber, T.X., and Calverley, D.S. Toward a theory of hypnotic behavior: Effects on suggestibility of task motivating instructions and attitudes toward hypnosis. *Journal of Abnormal and Social Psychology*, 1963, 67, 557-565. (c)

Barber, T.X., and Calverley, D.S. An experimental study of "hypnotic" (auditory and visual) hallucinations. *Journal of Abnormal and Social Psychology*, 1964, 63, 13-20. (a)

Barber, T.X., and Calverley, D.S. Effects of *E*'s tone of voice on "hypnotic-like" suggestibility. *Psychological Reports*, 1964, 15, 139-144. (b)

Barber, T.X., and Calverley, D.S. Empirical evidence for a theory of "hypnotic" behavior: Effects of pretest instructions on response to primary suggestions. *Psychological Record*, 1964, 14, 457-467. (c)

Barber, T.X., and Calverley, D.S. Experimental studies in "hypnotic" behavior: Suggested deafness evaluated by delayed auditory feedback. *British Journal of Psychology*, 1964, 55, 439-446. (d)

Barber, T.X., and Calverley, D.S. The definition of the situation as a variable affecting "hypnotic-like" suggestibility. *Journal of Clinical Psychology*, 1964, 20, 438-440. (e)

Barber, T.X., and Calverley, D.S. Toward a theory of hypnotic behavior: Effects on suggestibility of defining the situation as hypnosis and defining response to suggestions as easy. *Journal of Abnormal and Social Psychology*, 1964, 68, 585-592. (f)

Barber, T.X., and Calverley, D.S. Empirical evidence for a theory of "hypnotic" behavior: Effects on suggestibility of five variables typically included in hypnotic induction procedures. *Journal of Consulting Psychology*, 1965, 29, 98-107. (a)

Barber, T.X., and Calverley, D.S. Empirical evidence for a theory of "hypnotic" behavior: The suggestibility-enhancing effects of motivational suggestions, relaxation-sleep suggestions, and suggestions that the subject will be effectively "hypnotized." *Journal of Personality*, 1965, 33, 256-270. (b)

Barber, T.X., and Calverley, D.S. Effects on recall of hypnotic induction, motivational suggestions, and suggested regression: A methodological and experimental analysis. *Journal of Abnormal Psychology*, 1966, 71, 169-180. (a)

Barber, T.X., and Calverley, D.S. Toward a theory of "hypnotic" behavior: Experimental analyses of suggested amnesia. *Journal of Abnormal Psychology*, 1966, 71, 95-107. (b)

Barber, T.X., and Calverley, D.S. Toward a theory of hypnotic behavior: Experimental evaluation of Hull's postulate that hypnotic susceptibility is a habit phenomenon. *Journal of Personality*, 1966, 34, 416-433. (c)

Barber, T.X., and Calverley, D.S. Multidimensional analysis of "hypnotic" behavior. *Journal of Abnormal Psychology*, 1969, 74, 209-220.

Barber, T.X., and Cooper, B.J. Effects on pain of experimentally-induced and spontaneous distraction. *Psychological Reports*, 1972, 31, 647-651.

Barber, T.X., and Coules, J. Electrical skin conductance and galvanic skin response during "hypnosis." *International Journal of Clinical and Experimental Hypnosis*, 1959, 7, 79-92.

Barber, T.X., Dalal, A.S., and Calverley, D.S. The subjective reports of hypnotic subjects. *American Journal of Clinical Hypnosis*, 1968, 11, 74-88.

Barber, T.X., and Deeley, D.S. Experimental evidence for a theory of hypnotic behavior: I. "Hypnotic" color-blindness without "hypnosis." *International Journal of Clinical and Experimental Hypnosis*, 1961, 9, 79-86.

Barber, T.X., and DeMoor, W. A theory of hypnotic induction procedures. *American Journal of Clinical Hypnosis*, 1972, 15, 112-135.

Barber, T.X., DiCara, L.V., Kamiya, J., Miller, N.E., Shapiro, D., and Stoyva, J. (Eds.) *Biofeedback and Self-Control: 1970*. Chicago: Aldine-Atherton, 1971. (a)

Barber, T.X., DiCara, L.V., Kamiya, J., Miller, N.E., Shapiro, D., and Stoyva, J. *Biofeedback and Self-Control: An Aldine Reader on the Regulation of Bodily Processes and Consciousness*. Chicago: Aldine-Atherton, 1971. (b)

Barber, T.X. and Glass, L.B. Significant factors in hypnotic behavior. *Journal of Abnormal and Social Psychology*, 1962, 64, 222-228.

Barber, T.X., and Hahn, K.W., Jr. Physiological and subjective responses to pain producing stimulation under hypnotically-suggested and waking-imagined "analgesia." *Journal of Abnormal and Social Psychology*, 1962, 65, 411-418.

Barber, T.X., and Hahn, K.W., Jr. Hypnotic induction and "relaxation": An experimental study. *Archives of General Psychiatry*, 1963, 8, 295-300.

Barber, T.X., and Hahn, K.W., Jr. Suggested dreaming with and without hypnotic induction. Medfield, Mass.: Medfield Foundation, 1966. (Mimeo.)

Barber, T.X., and Silver, M.J. Fact, fiction, and the experimenter bias effect. *Psychological Bulletin (Monograph Supplement)*, 1968, 70 (6, Pt. 2), 1-29. (a)

Barber, T.X., and Silver, M.J. Pitfalls in data analysis and interpretation: A reply to Rosenthal. *Psychological Bulletin (Monograph Supplement)*, 1968, 70, (6, Pt. 2), 48-62. (b)

Barrett, C.L. Systematic desensitization versus implosive therapy. *Journal of Abnormal Psychology*, 1969, 74, 587-592.

Beecher, H.K. Pain in men wounded in battle. *Annals of Surgery*, 1946, 123, 96-105.

Beecher, H.K. The powerful placebo. *Journal of the American Medical Association*, 1955, 159, 1602-1606.

Beecher, H.K. Relationship of significance of wound to pain experienced. *Journal of the American Medical Association*, 1956, 161, 1609-1613.

Beecher, H.K. *Measurement of Subjective Responses*. New York: Oxford University Press, 1959.

Best, H.L., and Michaels, R.M. Living out "future" experience under hypnosis. *Science*, 1954, 120, 1077.

Betcher, A.M. Hypnosis as an adjunct in anesthesiology. *New York State Journal of Medicine*, 1960, 60, 816-822.

Binet, A., and Feré, C.S. *Animal Magnetism*. New York: Appleton, 1888.

Bloch, B. Ueber die Heilung der Warzen durch Suggestion. *Klinische Wochenschrift*, 1927, 6, 2271-2275, 2320-2325.

Blum, G.S. *A Model of the Mind*. New York: Wiley, 1961.

Blum, G.S., and Graef, J.R. The detection over time of subjects simulating hypnosis. *International Journal of Clinical and Experimental Hypnosis*, 1971, 19, 211-224.

Bonjour, J. Influence of the mind on the skin. *British Journal of Dermatology*, 1929, 41, 324-326.

Bowers, K.S. The effect of demands for honesty on reports of visual and auditory hallucinations. *International Journal of Clinical and Experimental Hypnosis*, 1967, 15, 31-36.

Braid, J. Facts and observations as to the relative value of mesmeric and hypnotic coma, and ethereal narcotism, for the mitigation or entire prevention of pain during surgical operations. *Medical Times*, 1847, 15, 381-382.

Bramwell, J.M. *Hypnotism*. New York: Julian Press, 1956. (Original date of publication: 1903.)

Brown, B.H. Cognitive aspects of Wolpe's Behavior Therapy. *American Journal of Psychiatry*, 1967, 124, 854-859.

Brown, P.E. Use of acupuncture in major surgery. *Lancet*, 1972, 1, 1328-1330.

Brown, R.A., Fader, K., and Barber, T.X. Responsiveness to pain: Stimulus-specificity versus generality. *Psychological Record*, 1973, 23, 1-7.

Bullard, P.D. The role of verbal reinforcement in hypnosis. *Journal of General Psychology*, 1973, 88, 141-149.

Burr, C.W. The reflexes of early infancy. *British Journal of Childhood Diseases*, 1921, 18, 152-153.

Capperauld, I. Acupuncture anesthesia and medicine in China today. *Surgery, Gynecology and Obstetrics*, 1972, 135, 440-445.

Cattell, M. The action and use of analgesics. *Research Publications Association for Research in Nervous and Mental Disease*, 1943, 23, 365-372.

Cautela, J.R. Covert extinction. *Behavior Therapy*, 1971, 2, 192-200.

Chaves, J.F. Hypnosis reconceptualized: An overview of Barber's theoretical and empirical work. *Psychological Reports*, 1968, 22, 587-608. [Reprinted in T.X. Barber et al. (Eds.) *Biofeedback and Self-Control: An Aldine Reader*. Chicago: Aldine-Atherton, 1971. Pp. 702-723.]

Chaves, J.F. Acupuncture analgesia: New data for psychology and psychophysiology. Paper presented at the annual meeting of the Massachusetts Psychological Association, Boston, May 12, 1972.

Chaves, J.F., and Barber, T.X. Needles and knives: Behind the mystery of acupuncture and Chinese meridians. *Human Behavior*, September 1973, 2, No. 9, 19-24.

Chaves, J.F., and Barber, T.X. Cognitive strategies, experimenter modeling, and expectation in the attenuation of pain. *Journal of Abnormal Psychology*, in press.

Chen, J.Y.P. Acupuncture. In J.R. Quinn (Ed.) *Medicine and Public Health in the People's Republic of China*. Washington, D.C.: U.S. Department of Health, Education, and Welfare, National Institutes of Health, 1972. Pp. 65-90.

Chertok, L. *Psychosomatic Methods in Painless Childbirth*. New York: Pergamon, 1959.

Chertok, L., and Kramarz, P. Hypnosis, sleep, and electro-encephalography. *Journal of Nervous and Mental Disease*, 1959, 128, 227-238.

Clarke, G.H.V. The charming of warts. *Journal of Investigative Dermatology*, 1965, 45, 15-21.

Coe, W.C. The heuristic value of role theory and hypnosis. Doctoral dissertation, University of California, Berkeley, 1964.

Coe, W.C., Allen, J.L., Krug, W.M., and Wurzmann, A.G. Goal-directed fantasy in difficult hypnotic items: Skill, item wording, or both. Department of Psychology, Fresno State University, 1972. (Mimeo.)

Collins, J.K. Muscular endurance in normal and hypnotic states: A study of suggested catalepsy. Honors thesis, Department of Psychology, University of Sydney, 1961.

Comins, J., Fullam, F., and Barber, T.X. Experimenter modeling, demands for honesty, and response to "hypnotic" suggestions. Medfield, Mass.: Medfield Foundation, 1973. (Mimeo.)

Conn, J.H., and Conn, R.N. Discussion of T.X. Barber's "Hypnosis as a causal variable in present-day psychology: A critical analysis." *International Journal of Clinical and Experimental Hypnosis*, 1967, 15, 106-110.

Cooper, L.M., Banford, S.A., Schubot, E., and Tart, C.T. A further attempt to modify hypnotic susceptibility through repeated individualized experience. *International Journal of Clinical and Experimental Hypnosis*, 1967, 15, 118-134.

Cooper, L.M., and Morgan, A.H. Accuracy of specific days given during hypnotic age regression. Stanford University: Hawthorne House Research Memorandum, #44, 1966. (Referred to by permission.)

Cooper, S.R., and Powles, W.E. The psychosomatic approach in practice. *McGill Medical Journal*, 1945, 14, 415-438.

Coppolino, C.A. *Practice of Hypnosis in Anesthesiology*. New York: Grune & Stratton, 1965.

Crasilneck, H.B., and Hall, J.A. Physiological changes associated with hypnosis: A review of the literature since 1948. *International Journal of Clinical and Experimental Hypnosis*, 1959, 7, 9-50.

Crasilneck, H.B., and Michael, C.M. Performance on the Bender under hypnotic age regression. *Journal of Abnormal and Social Psychology*, 1957, 54, 319-322.

Crasilneck, H.B., McCranie, E.J., and Jenkins, M.T. Special indications for hypnosis as a method of anesthesia. *Journal of the American Medical Association*, 1956, 162, 1606-1608.

Cronin, D.M., Spanos, N.P., and Barber, T.X. Augmenting hypnotic suggestibility by providing favorable information about hypnosis. *American Journal of Clinical Hypnosis*, 1971, 13, 259-264.

Dalal, A.S. An empirical approach to hypnosis: An overview of Barber's work. *Archives of General Psychiatry*, 1966, 15, 151-157.

Darnton, R. *Mesmerism and the End of the Enlightenment in France*. Cambridge, Mass.: Harvard University Press, 1968.

Dermen, D., and London, P. Correlates of hypnotic susceptibility. *Journal of Consulting Psychology*, 1965, 29, 537-545.

DeStefano, M.G. The modeling of hypnotic behavior. Doctoral dissertation, University of Montana, 1971.

De Voge, J.T., and Sachs, L.B. *The modification of hypnotic susceptibility through imitative behavior*. Paper presented at the annual meeting of the Southeastern Psychological Association, Miami, April 1971.

Diamond, M.J. The use of observationally-presented information to modify hypnotic susceptibility. *Journal of Abnormal Psychology*, 1972, 79, 174-180.

Diamond, M.J., Gregory, J., Lenney, E., Steadman, C., and Talone, J. Personality and hypnosis: The role of hypnosis-specific mediational attitudes in predicting hypnotic responsivity. *Proceedings, 80th Annual Convention, American Psychological Association*, 1972, 865-866.

Dimond, E.G. Acupuncture anesthesia: Western medicine and Chinese traditional medicine. *Journal of the American Medical Association*, 1971, 218, 1558-1563.

Dorcus, R.M., Brintnall, A.K., and Case, H.W. Control experiments and their relation to theories of hypnotism. *Journal of General Psychology*, 1941, 24, 217-221.

Doupe, J., Miller, W.R., and Keller, W.K. Vasomotor reactions in the hypnotic state. *Journal of Neurology and Psychiatry*, 1939, 2, 97-106.

Drake, D. Yin, Yang, and acupuncture. In *Acupuncture: What Can It Do for You?* New York: Newspaper Enterprise Association, 1972. Pp. 28-31.

Dudek, S.Z. Suggestion and play therapy in the cure of warts in children: A pilot study. *Journal of Nervous and Mental Disease*, 1967, 145, 37-42.

Dynes, J.B. An experimental study of hypnotic anesthesia. *Journal of Abnormal and Social Psychology*, 1932, 27, 79-88.

Edwards, A.L. *Techniques of Attitude Scale Construction*. New York: Appleton-Century-Crofts, 1957.

Egbert, L.D., Battit, G.E., Turndorf, H., and Beecher, H.K. The value of the preoperative visit by an anesthetist. *Journal of the American Medical Association*, 1963, 185, 553-555.

Egbert, L.D., Battit, G.E., Welch, C.E., and Bartlett, M.K. Reduction of postoperative pain by encouragement and instruction of patients. *New England Journal of Medicine*, 1964, 270, 825-827.

Erickson, M.H. A study of clinical and experimental findings on hypnotic deafness: I. Clinical experimentation and findings. *Journal of General Psychology*, 1938, 19, 127-150.

Erickson, M.H. The induction of color blindness by a technique of hypnotic suggestion. *Journal of General Psychology*, 1939, 20, 61-89.

Erickson, M.H. *Advanced Techniques of Hypnosis and Therapy*. (Edited by J. Haley.) New York: Grune & Stratton, 1967.

Esdaile, J. *Hypnosis in Medicine and Surgery*. New York: Julian Press, 1957. (Original date of publication: 1850.)

Estabrooks, G.H. *Hypnotism*. New York: E. P. Dutton, 1943.

Evans, F.J., and Orne, M.T. The disappearing hypnotist: The use of simulating subjects to evaluate how subjects perceive experimental procedures. *International Journal of Clinical and Experimental Hypnosis*, 1971, 19, 277-296.

Evans, M.B., and Paul, G.L. Effects of hypnotically suggested analgesia on physiological and subjective responses to cold stress. *Journal of Consulting and Clinical Psychology*, 1970, 35, 362-371. [Reprinted in J. Stoyva et al. (Ed.) *Biofeedback and Self-Control: 1971*. Chicago: Aldine-Atherton, 1972. Pp. 380-389.]

Finer, B.L. Experience with hypnosis in clinical anesthesiology. *Särtryck ur Opuscula Medica*, 1966, 4, 1-11.

Finer, B.L., and Nylen, B.O. Cardiac arrest in the treatment of burns, and report on hypnosis as a substitute for anesthesia. *Plastic and Reconstructive Surgery*, 1961, 27, 49-55.

Fisher, S. Problems of interpretation and controls in hypnotic research. In G.H. Estabrooks (Ed.) *Hypnosis: Current Problems*. New York: Harper & Row, 1962. Pp. 109-126.

Forgione, A.G., and Barber, T.X. A strain gauge pain stimulator. *Psychophysiology*, 1971, 8, 102-106.

Foulkes, D. *The Psychology of Sleep*. New York: Charles Scribner's, 1966.

Franks, C.M. (Ed.) *Behavior Therapy: Appraisal and Status*. New York: McGraw-Hill, 1969.

Freedman, L.R. The relevance of acupuncture. *Yale Journal of Biology and Medicine*, 1972, 45, 70-72.

Freemont-Smith, F. Discussion of Beecher's paper on perception of pain. Problems of Consciousness, First Conference. New York: Josiah Macy, Jr. Foundation, 1950.

Fromm, E., and R.E. Shor (Eds.) *Hypnosis: Research Developments and Perspectives*. Chicago: Aldine-Atherton, 1972.

Gammon, G.D., and Starr, I. Studies on the relief of pain by counterirritation. *Journal of Clinical Investigation*, 1941, 20, 13-20.

Gammon, G.D., Starr, I., and Bronk, D.W. The effect of counterirritation upon pain produced by cutaneous injury. *American Journal of Physiology*, 1936, 116, 56.

Gidro-Frank, L., and Bowersbuch, M.K. A study of the plantar response in hypnotic age regression. *Journal of Nervous and Mental Disease*, 1948, 107, 443-458.

Gill, M.M., and Brenman, M. *Hypnosis and Related States*. New York: International Universities Press, 1959.

Gindes, B.C. *New Concepts of Hypnosis*. New York: Julian Press, 1951.

Gordon, J.E., and Freston, M. Role-playing and age regression in hypnotized and non-hypnotized subjects. *Journal of Personality*, 1964, 32, 411-419.

Graham, C., and Leibowitz, H.W. The effect of suggestion on visual acuity. *International Journal of Clinical and Experimental Hypnosis*, 1972, 20, 169-186.

Green, E.E., Ferguson, D.W., Green, A.M., and Walters, E.D. Preliminary report on voluntary controls project: Swami Rama. Topeka: Menninger Foundation, 1970.

Green, E.E., Green, A.M., and Walters, E.D. Voluntary control of internal states: Psychological and physiological. *Journal of Transpersonal Psychology*, 1970, 2, 1-26.

Green, E.E., Walters, E.D., Green, A.M., and Murphy, G. Feedback technique for deep relaxation. *Psychophysiology*, 1969, 6, 371-377. [Reprinted in T.X. Barber et al. (Eds.) *Biofeedback and Self-Control: An Aldine Reader*. Chicago: Aldine-Atherton, 1971. Pp. 402-409.]

Greenberg, R.P., and Land, J.M. Influence of some hypnotist and subject variables on hypnotic susceptibility. *Journal of Consulting and Clinical Psychology*, 1971, 37, 111-115.

Greenleaf, E. Developmental-stage regression through hypnosis. *American Journal of Clinical Hypnosis*, 1969, 12, 20-36.

Gregory, J., and Diamond, M.J. Increasing hypnotic susceptibility by means of positive expectancies and writen instructions. *Journal of Abnormal Psychology*, 1973, 82, 363-367.

Hadfield, J.A. The influence of suggestion on body temperature. *Lancet*, 1920, 2, 68-69.

Harano, K., Ogawa, K., and Naruse, G. A study of plethysmography and skin temperature during active concentration and autogenic exercise. In W. Luthe (Ed.) *Autogenic Training*. New York: Grune & Stratton, 1965. Pp. 55-58.

Hardy, J.D., Wolff, H.G., and Goodell, H. *Pain Sensations and Reactions*. Baltimore: Williams & Wilkins, 1952.

Hartland, J. *Medical and Dental Hypnosis and its Clinical Applications*. Baltimore: Williams & Wilkins, 1966, Second Edition–London: Baillière Tindall, 1971.

Harwood, L.W. Changes in visual acuity in myopic subjects during hypnosis. Paper presented at the annual meeting of the American Academy of Optometry, Miami, December 13, 1970.

Harwood, L.R. Changes in visual acuity in myopic subjects which are similar to those in hypnotized myopic subjects. Paper presented at the annual meeting of the American Academy of Optometry, Toronto, 1971.

Hendin, D. Is acupuncture today's medical miracle? In *Acupuncture: What Can It Do for You?* New York: Newspaper Enterprise Association, 1972. Pp. 4-7.

Hilgard, E.R. *Hypnotic Susceptibility*. New York: Harcourt Brace Jovanovich, 1965.

Hilgard, E.R. Posthypnotic amnesia: Experiments and theory. *International Journal of Clinical and Experimental Hypnosis*, 1966, 14, 104-111.

Hilgard, E.R. A quantitative study of pain and its reduction through hypnotic suggestion. *Proceedings of the National Academy of Science*, 1967, 57, 1581-1586.

Hilgard, E.R. Altered states of awareness. *Journal of Nervous and Mental Disease*, 1969, 149, 68-79. (a) [Reprinted in T.X. Barber et al. (Eds.) *Biofeedback and Self-Control:*

An Aldine Reader. Chicago: Aldine-Atherton, 1971. Pp. 763-774.]

Hilgard, E.R. Pain as a puzzle for psychology and physiology. *American Psychologist*, 1969, 24, 103-113. (b)

Hilgard, E.R. A critique of Johnson, Maher, and Barber's "Artifact in the 'essence of hypnosis': An evaluation of trance logic," with a recomputation of their findings. *Journal of Abnormal Psychology*, 1972, 79, 221-233.

Hilgard, E.R., Cooper, L.M., Lenox, J., Morgan, A.H., and Voevodsky, J. The use of pain-state reports in the study of hypnotic analgesia to the pain of ice water. *Journal of Nervous and Mental Disease*, 1967, 144, 506-513.

Hilgard, J.R. *Personality and Hypnosis.* Chicago: University of Chicago Press, 1970.

Hilgard, J.R., and Hilgard, E.R. Developmental-interactive aspects of hypnosis: Some illustrative cases. *Genetic Psychology Monographs*, 1962, 66, 143-178.

Hill, H.E., Kornetsky, C.H., Flanary, H.G., and Wikler, A. Effects of anxiety and morphine on discrimination of intensities of painful stimuli. *Journal of Clinical Investigation*, 1952, 31, 473-480. (a)

Hill, H.E., Kornetsky, C.H., Flanary, H.G., and Wikler, A. Studies on anxiety associated with anticipation of pain. I. Effects of morphine. *Archives of Neurology and Psychiatry*, 1952, 67, 612-619. (b)

Hoffman, E. Hypnosis in general surgery. *American Surgeon*, 1959, 25, 163-169.

Hoskovec, J., and Horvai, I. Speech manifestations in hypnotic age regression. *Activitas nervosa superior*, 1963, 5, 13-21.

Houde, R.W., and Wallenstein, S.L. A method for evaluating analgesics in patients with chronic pain. *Drug Addiction and Narcotics, Bulletin*, 1953, Appendix F, 660-682.

Hull, C.L. *Hypnosis and Suggestibility: An Experimental Approach.* New York: Appleton-Century, 1933.

Ikemi, Y. Hypnotic experiments on the psychosomatic aspects of gastrointestinal disorders. *International Journal of Clinical and Experimental Hypnosis*, 1959, 7, 139-150.

Ikemi, Y., and Nakagawa, S. A psychosomatic study of contagious dermatitis. *Kyushu Journal of Medical Science*, 1962, 13, 335-350.

Jacobson, A., Kales, A., Lehmann, D., and Zweizig, J.R. Somnambulism: All-night electroencephalographic studies. *Science*, 1965, 148, 975-977.

Jacobson, E. Electrical measurements of neuromuscular states during mental activities. *American Journal of Physiology*, 1930, 91, 567.

Jacobson, E. Electrophysiology of mental activities. *American Journal of Psychology*, 1932, 44, 677-694.

Johnson, R.F.Q. Trance logic revisited: A reply to Hilgard's critique. *Journal of Abnormal Psychology*, 1972, 79, 234-238.

Johnson, R.F.Q., Maher, B.A., and Barber, T.X. Artifact in the "essence of hypnosis": An evaluation of trance logic. *Journal of Abnormal Psychology*, 1972, 79, 212-220.

Juhasz, J.B. Imagination, imitation, and role taking. Ann Arbor, Michigan: University Microfilms, 70-13, 076, 1969.

Kales, A., Jacobson, A., Paulson, M.J., Kales, J.D., and Walter, R.D. Somnambulism: Psychophysiological correlates. I. All-night EEG studies. *Archives of General Psychiatry*, 1966, 14, 586-594.

Kanfer, F.H., and Goldfoot, D.A. Self-control and tolerance of noxious stimulation. *Psychological Reports*, 1966, 18, 79-85.

Keats, A.S. Postoperative pain: Research and treatment. *Journal of Chronic Diseases*, 1956, 4, 72-80.

Kelley, C.R. Psychological factors in myopia. Doctoral dissertation, New School for Social Research, 1958. .

Kelley, C.R. Psychological factors in myopia. Paper presented at the annual meeting of the American Psychological Association, New York, August 31, 1961.

Kiesler, C.A., Collins, B.E., and Miller, N. *Attitude Change: A Critical Analysis of Theoretical Approaches.* New York: Wiley, 1969.

Kinney, J.C.M. Modification of hypnotic susceptibility. Doctoral dissertation, Stanford University, 1969. Ann Arbor, Michigan: University Microfilms, 70-10, 476.

Klein, M.H., Dittman, A.T., Parloff, M.B., and Gill, M.M. Behavior therapy: Observations and reflections. *Journal of Consulting and Clinical Psychology*, 1969, 33, 259-266.

Klemme, H.L. Heart rate response to suggestion in hypnosis. Topeka: Veterans Administration Hospital, 1963. (Mimeo.)

Kline, M.V. Hypnosis and age progression: A case report. *Journal of Genetic Psychology*, 1951, 78, 195-208.

Kline, M.V., Guze, H., and Haggerty, A.D. An experimental study of the nature of hypnotic deafness: Effects of delayed speech feedback. *Journal of Clinical and Experimental Hypnosis*, 1954, 2, 145-156.

Klinger, B.I. Effect of peer model responsiveness and length of induction procedure on hypnotic responsiveness. *Journal of Abnormal Psychology*, 1970, 75, 15-18.

Klopp, K.K. Production of local anesthesia using waking suggestion with the child patient. *International Journal of Clinical and Experimental Hypnosis*, 1961, 9, 59-62.

Kornetsky, C. Effects of anxiety and morphine in the anticipation and perception of painful radiant heat stimuli. *Journal of Comparative and Physiological Psychology*, 1954, 47, 130-132.

Kramer, E. Hypnotic susceptibility and previous relationship with the hypnotist. *American Journal of Clinical Hypnosis*, 1969, 11, 175-177.

Kramer, E., and Tucker, G.R. Hypnotically suggested deafness and delayed auditory feedback. *International Journal of Clinical and Experimental Hypnosis*, 1967, 15, 37-43.

Kroger, W.S. Introduction and supplemental reports. In J. Esdaile, *Hypnosis in Medicine and Surgery.* New York: Julian Press, 1957.

Kroger, W.S. Hypnotism and acupuncture. *Journal of the American Medical Association*, 1972, 220, 1012-1013. (a)

Kroger, W.S. More on acupuncture and hypnosis. *Society for Clinical and Experimental Hypnosis Newsletter*, 1972, 13, No. 4, 2-3. (b)

Kroger, W.S., and DeLee, S.T. Use of hypnoanaesthesia for cesarean section and hysterectomy. *Journal of the American Medical Association*, 1957, 163, 442-444.

Lasagna, L., Mosteller, F., von Felsinger, J.M., and Beecher, H.K. A study of the placebo response. *American Journal of Medicine*, 1954, 16, 770-779.

Lassner, J. (Ed.) *Hypnosis in Anesthesiology.* Berlin: Springer-Verlag, 1964.

Laszlo, D., and Spencer, H. Medical problems in the management of cancer. *Medical Clinics of North America*, 1953, 37, 869-880.

Lazarus, A.A. *Behavior Therapy and Beyond.* New York: McGraw-Hill, 1971.

Lee-Teng, E. Trance-susceptibility, induction-susceptibility, and acquiescence as factors in hypnotic performance. *Journal of Abnormal Psychology*, 1965, 70, 383-389.

Leitenberg, H., Agras, W.S., Barlow, D.H., and Oliveau, D.C. Contribution of selective positive reinforcement and therapeutic instructions to systematic desensitization therapy. *Journal of Abnormal Psychology*, 1969, 74, 113-118.

Lennander, K.G. Ueber die Sensibilität der Bauchhöhle und über lokale und allgemeine Anästhesie bei Bruch-und Bauchoperationen. *Centralblatt für Chirurgie*, 1901, 8, 209-223.

Lennander, K.G. Beobachtungen über die Sensibilität in der Bauchhöhle. *Mitteilungen aus den Grenzgebieten der Medizin und Chirurgie*, 1902, 10, 38-104.

Lennander, K.G. Weitere Beobachtungen über Sensibilität in Organ und Gewebe und über lokale Anästhesie. *Deutsche Zeitschrift für Chirurgie*, 1904, 73, 297-350.

Lennander, K.G. Ueber Hofrat Nothnagels zweite Hypothese der Darmkolikschmerzen. *Mitteilungen aus den Grenzgebieten der Medizin und Chirurgie*, 1906, 16, 19-23. (a)

Lennander, K.G. Ueber lokale Anästhesie und uber Sensibilität in Organ und Gewebe, weitere Beobachtungen. *Mitteilungen aus den Grenzgebieten der Medizin und Chirurgie*, 1906, 15, 465-494. (b)

Leonard, J.R. An investigation of hypnotic age-regression. Doctoral dissertation, University of Kentucky, 1963.

Leonard, J.R. Hypnotic age-regression: A test of the functional ablation hypothesis. *Journal of Abnormal Psychology*, 1965, 70, 266-269.

Levine, M. Psychogalvanic reaction to painful stimuli in hypnotic and hysterical anesthesia. *Bulletin of the Johns Hopkins Hospital*, 1930, 46, 331-339.

Levitt, E.E., and Brady, J.P. Psychophysiology of hypnosis. In J.M. Schneck (Ed.) *Hypnosis in Modern Medicine*. (3rd Ed.) Springfield, Ill.: C.C. Thomas, 1963. Pp. 314-362.

Lewis, I.M. *Ecstatic Religion: An Anthropological Study of Spirit Possession and Shamanism*. Baltimore: Penguin, 1971.

Lewis, J.H., and Sarbin, T.R. Studies in psychosomatics: I. The influence of hypnotic stimulation on gastric hunger contractions. *Psychosomatic Medicine*, 1943, 5, 125-131.

Lewis, T. *Pain*. New York: Macmillan, 1942.

Liebeault, A.A. Anesthesia per suggestion. *Journal Magnestisme*, 1885, 64-67.

Liu, W. Acupuncture anesthesia: A case report. *Journal of the American Medical Association*, 1972, 221, 87-88.

London, P. Subject characteristics in hypnosis research: I. A survey of experience, interest, and opinion. *International Journal of Clinical and Experimental Hypnosis*, 1961, 9, 151-161.

London, P. The induction of hypnosis. In J.E. Gordon (Ed.) *Handbook of Clinical and Experimental Hypnosis*. New York: Macmillan, 1967. Pp. 44-79.

London, P., Cooper L.M., and Johnson, H.J. Subject characteristics in hypnosis research: II. Attitudes toward hypnosis, volunteer status, and personality measures.III. Some correlates of hypnotic susceptibility. *International Journal of Clinical and Experimental Hypnosis*, 1962, 10, 13-21.

Lonk, A.F. *A Manual of Hypnotism and Psycho-Therapeutics*. (Revised 3rd Ed.) Palatine, Ill.: Adolph F. Lonk, 1947.

Lozanov, G. Anaesthetization through suggestion in a state of wakefulness. *Proceedings of the 7th European Conference on Psychosomatic Research*, Rome, 1967, 399-402.

Luckhardt, A.B., and Johnston, R.L. Studies in gastric secretions: I. The psychic secretion of gastric juice under hypnosis. *American Journal of Physiology*, 1924, 70, 174-182.

Macvaugh, G.S. *Hypnosis Readiness Inventory*. Chevy Chase, Md.: G.S. Macvaugh (4402 Stanford Street), 1969.

Man, P.L., and Chen, C.H. Acupuncture "anesthesia"—a new theory and clinical study. *Current Therapeutic Research*, 1972, 14, 390-394.

Mandy, A.J., Mandy, T.E., Farkas, R., and Scher, E. Is natural childbirth natural? *Psychosomatic Medicine*, 1952, 14, 431-438.

Mann, F. *Acupuncture: The Ancient Chinese Art of Healing*. New York: Vintage Books, 1962.

Mann, F. The probable neurophysiological mechanism of acupuncture. In *Transcript of the Acupuncture Symposium*. Los Altos, Calif.: Academy of Parapsychology and Medicine, 1972. Pp. 24-31.

Mann, F. Paper presented at the New York University School of Medicine, Symposium on Acupuncture, 1973.

Marmer, M.J. The role of hypnosis in anesthesiology. *Journal of the American Medical Association*, 1956, 162, 441-443.

Marmer, M.J. Hypnoanalgesia: The use of hypnosis in conjunction with chemical anesthesia. *Anesthesia and Analgesia*, 1957, 36, 27-32.

Marmer, M.J. *Hypnosis in Anesthesiology*. Springfield, Ill.: C.C. Thomas, 1959.

Marshall, G., and Diamond, M.J. Increasing hypnotic behavior through modeling. Department of Psychology, Stanford University, 1968.

Mason, A.A. Surgery under hypnosis. *Anesthesia*, 1955, 10, 295-299.

Matheus, J.M. Effects on suggestibility of experimenter prestige under hypnotic induction, task motivation, and waking imagination conditions. *American Journal of Clinical Hypnosis*, 1973, 15, 199-208.

Matsumoto, T. Acupuncture and U.S. medicine. *Journal of the American Medical Association*, 1972, 220, 1010.

McGarey, W.A. The philosophy and clinical aspects of acupuncture as viewed from the framework of Western medicine. In *Transcript of the Acupuncture Symposium*. Los Altos, Calif.: Academy of Parapsychology and Medicine, 1972. Pp. 12-22.

McGill, O. *The Encyclopedia of Stage Hypnotism*. Colon, Mich.: Abbott's Magic Novelty Co., 1947.

McGuire, W.J. Personality and susceptibility to social influence. In E.F. Borgatta and W.W. Lambert (Eds.) *Handbook of Personality Theory and Research*. Chicago: Rand McNally, 1968. Pp. 1130-1187.

McPeake, J.D. Hypnosis, suggestions, and psychosomatics. *Diseases of the Nervous System*, 1968, 29, 536-544.

McPeake, J.D., and Spanos, N.P. The effects of the wording of rating scales on hypnotic subjects' descriptions of visual hallucinations. *American Journal of Clinical Hypnosis*, 1973, 15, 239-244.

Meeker, W.B., and Barber, T.X. Toward an explanation of stage hypnosis. *Journal of Abnormal Psychology*, 1971, 77, 61-70. [Reprinted in J. Stoyva et al. (Eds.) *Biofeedback and Self-Control: 1971*. Chicago: Aldine-Atherton, 1972. Pp. 395-404.]

Melei, J.P., and Hilgard, E.R. Attitudes toward hypnosis, self-predictions, and hypnotic susceptibility. *International Journal of Clinical and Experimental Hypnosis*, 1964, 12, 99-108.

Melzack, R. Why acupuncture works. *Psychology Today*, June 1973, 7. No. 1, 28-37.

Melzack, R., and Wall, P. Pain mechanisms: A new theory. *Science*, 1965, 150, 971-979.

Memmesheimer, A.M., and Eisenlohr, E. Untersuchungen über die Suggestivbehandlung der Warzen. *Dermatologie Zietschrift*, 1931, 62, 63-68.

Menzies, R. Further studies of conditioned vasomotor responses in human subjects. *Journal of Experimental Psychology*, 1941, 29, 457-482.

Mesel, E., and Ledford, F.F., Jr. The electroencephalogram during hypnotic age regression (to infancy) in epileptic patients. *Archives of Neurology*, 1959, 1, 516-521.

Miller, R. J., Bergeim, O., Rehfuss, M.E., and Hawk, P.B. Gastric response to food: X. The psychic secretion of gastric juice in normal men. *American Journal of Physiology*, 1920, 52, 1-27.

Miller, S.B. The contribution of therapeutic instructions to systematic desensitization. *Behavior Research and Therapy*, 1972, 10, 159-169.

Mitchell, J.F. Local anesthesia in general surgery. *Journal of the American Medical Association*, 1907, 48, 198-201.

Moll, A. *The Study of Hypnosis*. New York: Julian Press, 1958. (Original date of publication: 1889.)

Mordey, T.R. The relationship between certain motives and suggestibility. Masters thesis, Roosevelt University, 1960.

Morgan, A.H., Lezard, F., Prytulak, S., and Hilgard, E.R. Augmenters, reducers, and their reaction to cold pressor pain in waking and suggested hypnotic analgesia. *Journal of Personality and Social Psychology*, 1970, 16, 5-11.

Moss, C.S. *Hypnosis in Perspective*. New York: Macmillan, 1965.

Nace, E.P. and Orne, M.T. Fate of an uncompleted posthypnotic suggestion. *Journal of Abnormal Psychology*, 1970, 75, 278-285.

Nelson, R.A. *A Complete Course in Stage Hypnotism*. Columbus, Ohio: Nelson Enterprises, 1965.

Nichols, D.C. A reconceptualization of the concept of hypnosis. In S. Leese (Ed.) *An Evaluation of the Results of the Psychotherapies*. Springfield, Ill.: C.C. Thomas, 1968. Chap. 11.

Norris, D.L. Barber's task-motivational theory and post-hypnotic amnesia. *American Journal of Clinical Hypnosis*, 1973, 15, 181-190.

Notermans, S.L.H. Measurement of the pain threshold determined by electrical stimulation and its clinical application. Part I. Method and factors possibly influencing the pain threshold. *Neurology*, 1966, 16, 1071-1086.

Notermans, S.L.H. Measurement of the pain threshold determined by electrical stimulation and its clinical application. Part II. Clinical application in neurological and neurosurgical patients. *Neurology*, 1967, 17, 58-73.

O'Connell, D.N., Shor, R.E., and Orne, M.T. Hypnotic age regression: An empirical and methodological analysis. *Journal of Abnormal Psychology Monograph Supplement*, 1970, 76, No. 3, Part 2, 1-32.

Oliveau, D.C., Agras, W.S., Leitenberg, H., Moore, R.C., and Wright, D.E. Systematic desensitization, therapeutically oriented instructions and selective positive reinforcement. *Behaviour Research and Therapy*, 1969, 7, 27-33.

Orne, M.T. The mechanisms of hypnotic age regression: An experimental study. *Journal of Abnormal and Social Psychology*, 1951, 46, 213-225.

Orne, M.T. The nature of hypnosis: Artifact and essence. *Journal of Abnormal and Social Psychology*, 1959, 58, 277-299.

Orne, M.T. On the mechanism of posthypnotic amnesia. *International Journal of Clinical and Experimental Hypnosis*, 1966, 14, 121-134.

Orne, M.T., and Evans, F.J. Inadvertent termination of hypnosis with hypnotized and simulating objects. *International Journal of Clinical and Experimental Hypnosis*, 1966, 14, 61-78.

Orne, M.T., Sheehan, P.W., and Evans, F.J. Occurrence of posthypnotic behavior outside the experimental setting. *Journal of Personality and Social Psychology*, 1968, 9, 189-196.

Ostenasek, F.J. Prefrontal lobotomy for the relief of intractable pain. *Bulletin of the Johns Hopkins Hospital*, 1948, 83, 229-236.

Pai, M.N. Sleep-walking and sleep activities. *Journal of Mental Science*, 1946, 92, 756-783.

Parrish, M., Lundy, R.M., and Leibowitz, H.W. Effect of hypnotic age regression on the magnitude of the Ponzo and Poggendorff illusions. *Journal of Abnormal Psychology*, 1969, 74, 693-698.

Pattie, F.A. Methods of induction, susceptibility of subjects, and criteria of hypnosis. In R.M. Dorcus (Ed.) *Hypnosis and its Therapeutic Applications*. New York: McGraw-Hill, 1956. Chap. 2. (a)

Pattie, F.A. Theories of hypnosis. In R.M. Dorcus (Ed.) *Hypnosis and its Therapeutic Applications*. New York: McGraw-Hill, 1956. Chap. 1. (b)

Perry, C., and Chisholm. W. Hypnotic age regression and the Ponzo and Poggendorff illusions. *International Journal of Clinical and Experimental Hypnosis*, 1973, 21, 192-204.

Porter, J.W., Woodward, J.A., Bisbee, T.C., and Fenker, R.M., Jr. Effect of hypnotic age regression on the magnitude of the Ponzo illusion. *Journal of Abnormal Psychology*, 1971, 79, 189-194.

Powers, E.M. The effect of experimenter attitude, type of instruction, and method of presentation on the performance of hypnotic behavior. Masters thesis, University of New Hampshire, 1972.

Ratner, S.C. Comparative aspects of hypnosis. In J.E. Gordon (Ed.) *Handbook of Clinical and Experimental Hypnosis*. New York: Macmillan, 1967. Pp. 550-587.

Rechtschaffen, A., Vogel, G., and Shaikun, G. Interrelatedness of mental activity during sleep. *Archives of General Psychiatry*, 1963, 9, 536-547.

Reiff, R., and Scheerer, H. *Memory and Hypnotic Age Regression*. New York: International Universities Press, 1959.

Reis, M. Subjective reactions of a patient having surgery without chemical anesthesia. *American Journal of Clinical Hypnosis*, 1966, 9, 122-124.

Reston, J. Now, about my operation. *In Acupuncture: What Can It Do for You?* New York: Newspaper Enterprise Association, 1972. Pp. 8-11.

Rhee, J.L. Introductory remarks: "Acupuncture: The need for an in depth appraisal." *In Transcript of the Acupuncture Symposium*. Los Altos, Calif.: Academy of Parapsychology and Medicine, 1972. Pp. 8-10

Richman, D.N. A critique of two recent theories of hypnosis: The psychoanalytic theory of Gill and Brenman contrasted with the behavioral theory of Barber. *Psychiatric Quarterly*, 1965, 39, 278-292.

Roberts, A.H., Kewman, D.G., and MacDonald, H. Voluntary control of skin temperature: Unilateral changes using hypnosis and feedback. *Journal of Abnormal Psychology*, 1973, 82, 163-168.

Rosenberg, M.J. A disconfirmation of the description of hypnosis as a dissociated state. *International Journal of Clinical and Experimental Hypnosis*, 1959, 7, 187-204.

Rosenhan, D.L., and Tomkins, S.S. On preference for hypnosis and hypnotizability. *International Journal of Clinical and Experimental Hypnosis*, 1964, 12, 109-114.

Rosenthal, R. Experimenter expectancy and the reassuring nature of the null hypothesis decision procedure. *Psychological Bulletin Monograph*, 1968, 70, (6, Pt. 2), 30-47.

Rubenstein, R., and Newman, R. The living out of "future" experiences under hypnosis. *Science*, 1954, 119, 472-473.

Sachs, L.B. Modification of hypnotic behavior without hypnotic inductions. Department of Psychology, West Virginia University, 1969.

Sachs, L.B. Construing hypnosis as modifiable behavior. In A. Jacobs and L.B. Sachs (Eds.) *The Psychology of Private Events.* New York: Academic Press, 1971. Pp. 61-75.

Sachs, L.B., and Anderson, W.L. Modification of hypnotic susceptibility. *International Journal of Clinical and Experimental Hypnosis*, 1967, 15, 172-180.

Sampimon, R.L.H., and Woodruff, M.F.A. Some observations concerning the use of hypnosis as a substitute for anesthesia. *Medical Journal of Australia*, 1946, 1, 393-395.

Sarbin, T.R. Contributions to role-taking theory: I. Hypnotic behavior. *Psychological Review*, 1950, 57, 255-270. (a).

Sarbin, T.R. Mental changes in experimental regression. *Journal of Personality*, 1950, 19, 221-228. (b)

Sarbin, T.R. Physiological effects of hypnotic stimulation. In R.M. Dorcus (Ed.) *Hypnosis and its Therapeutic Applications.* New York: McGraw-Hill, 1956. Chap. 4.

Sarbin, T.R. Imagining as muted role-taking: A historical-linguistic analysis. In P.W. Sheehan (Ed.) *The Function and Nature of Imagery.* New York: Academic Press, 1972. Pp. 333-354.

Sarbin, T.R., and Andersen, M.L. Role-theoretical analysis of hypnotic behavior. In J.E. Gordon (Ed.) *Handbook of Clinical and Experimental Hypnosis.* New York: Macmillan, 1967. Pp. 319-344.

Sarbin, T.R., and Coe, W.C. *Hypnosis: A Social Psychological Analysis of Influence Communication.* New York: Holt, Rinehart, & Winston, 1972.

Sarbin, T.R., and Farberow, N.L. Contributions to role-taking theory: A clinical study of self and role. *Journal of Abnormal and Social Psychology*, 1952, 47, 117-125.

Sarbin, T.R., and Juhasz, J.B. Toward a theory of imagination. *Journal of Personality*, 1970, 38, 52-76.

Sarbin, T.R., and Slagle, R.W. Hypnosis and psychophysiological outcomes. In E. Fromm and R.E. Shor (Eds.) *Hypnosis: Research Developments and Perspectives* Chicago: Aldine-Atherton, 1972. Pp. 185-214.

Sattler, D.G. Absence of local sign in visceral reactions to painful stimulation. *Research Publications Association for Research in Nervous and Mental Disease*, 1943, 23, 143-153.

Scheibe, K.E., Gray, A.L., and Keim, C.S. Hypnotically induced deafness and delayed auditory feedback: A comparison of real and simulating subjects. *International Journal of Clinical and Experimental Hypnosis*, 1968, 16, 158-164.

Schneck, J.M. Relationship between hypnotist-audience and hypnotist-subject interaction. *Journal of Clinical and Experimental Hypnosis*, 1958, 6, 171-181.

Schneck, J.M. *Principles and Practice of Hypnoanalysis.* Springfield, Ill.: C.C. Thomas, 1965.

Schultz, J.H. Ueber selbsttätige (autogene) Umstellungen der Wärmestrahlung der Menschlichen Haut im Autosuggestiven Training. *Deutsche medizinische Wochenschrift*, 1926, 14, 571-572.

Schultz, J.H. *Das Autogene Training.* Leipzig: G. Thieme Verlag, 1932.

Schwarcz, B.E. Hypnoanalgesia and hypnoanesthesia in urology. *Surgical Clinics of North America*, 1965, 45, 7547-7555.

Secord, P.F., and Backman, C.W. *Social Psychology*. New York: McGraw-Hill, 1964.

Shealy, C.N. A physiological basis for electro-acupuncture. In *Transcript of the Acupuncture Symposium*. Los Altos, Calif.: Academy of Parapsychology and Medicine, 1972, Pp. 34-36.

Sheehan, P.W., and Orne, M.T. Some comments on the nature of posthypnotic behavior. *Journal of Nervous and Mental Disease*, 1968, 148, 209-220.

Shor, R.E. The three-factor theory of hypnosis as applied to the book-reading fantasy and to the concept of suggestion. *International Journal of Clinical and Experimental Hypnosis*, 1970, 18, 89-98.

Shor, R.E., Expectancies of being influenced and hypnotic performance. *International Journal of Clinical and Experimental Hypnosis*, 1971, 19, 154-166.

Shor, R.E., and Orne, M.T. *The Nature of Hypnosis: Selected Basic Readings*. New York: Holt, Rinehart, & Winston, 1965.

Shor, R.E., Orne, M.T., and O'Connell, D.N. Validation and cross-validation of a scale of self-reported personal experiences which predicts hypnotizability. *Journal of Psychology*, 1962, 53, 55-75.

Shor, R.E., Orne, M.T., and O'Connell, D.N. Psychological correlates of plateau hypnotizability in a special volunteer sample. *Journal of Personality and Social Psychology*, 1966, 3, 80-95.

Sinclair-Gieben, A.H.C., and Chalmers, D. Evaluation of treatment of warts by hypnosis. *Lancet*, 1959, 2, 480-482.

Small, M.M., and Kramer, E. Hypnotic susceptibility as a function of the prestige of the hypnotist. *International Journal of Clinical and Experimental Hypnosis*, 1969, 17, 251-256.

Solomon, D., and Goodson, D.F. Hypnotic age regression evaluated against a criterion of prior performance. *International Journal of Clinical and Experimental Hypnosis*, 1971, 19, 243-259.

Spanos, N.P. Barber's reconceptualization of hypnosis: An evaluation of criticisms. *Journal of Experimental Research in Personality*, 1970, 4, 241-258. [Reprinted in J. Stoyva et al. (Eds.) *Biofeedback and Self-Control: 1971*. Chicago: Aldine-Atherton, 1972. Pp. 352-368.]

Spanos, N.P. Goal-directed phantasy and the performance of hypnotic test suggestions. *Psychiatry*, 1971, 34, 86-96.

Spanos, N.P., and Barber, T.X. "Hypnotic" experiences as inferred from subjective reports: Auditory and visual hallucinations. *Journal of Experimental Research in Personality*, 1968, 3, 136-150.

Spanos, N.P., and Barber, T.X. Cognitive activity during "hypnotic" suggestibility: Goal-directed fantasy and the experience of non-volition. *Journal of Personality*, 1972, 40, 510-524.

Spanos, N.P., and Barber, T.X. Book review: Orne's work on hypnosis. *American Journal of Clinical Hypnosis*, 1973, 16, 138-141.

Spanos, N.P., Barber, T.X., and Lang, G. Effects of hypnotic induction, suggestions of analgesia, and demands for honesty on subjective reports of pain. Department of Sociology, Boston University, 1969.

Spanos, N.P., and Chaves, J.F. Hypnosis research: A methodological critique of two alternative paradigms. *American Journal of Clinical Hypnosis*, 1970, 13, 108-127. [Reprinted in T.X. Barber et al. (Eds.) *Biofeedback and Self-Control: 1970*. Chicago: Aldine-Atherton, 1971. Pp. 168-187.]

Spanos, N.P., DeMoor, W., and Barber, T.X. Hypnosis and behavior therapy: Common denominators. *American Journal of Clinical Hypnosis*, 1973, 16, 45-64.

Spanos, N.P., and Ham, M.L. Cognitive activity in response to hypnotic suggestions: Goal-directed fantasy and selective amnesia. *American Journal of Clinical Hypnosis*, 1973, 15, 191-198.

Spanos, N.P., Ham, M.W., and Barber, T.X. Suggested ("hypnotic") visual hallucinations: Experimental and phenomenological data. *Journal of Abnormal Psychology*, 1973, 81, 96-106.

Spanos, N.P., and McPeake, J.D. Effect of attitudes toward hypnosis on the relationship between involvement in everyday imaginative activities and hypnotic suggestibility. Medfield, Mass.: Medfield Foundation, 1973. (a) (Mimeo.)

Spanos, N.P., and McPeake, J.D. Involvement in everyday imaginative activities, attitudes toward hypnosis, and hypnotic suggestibility. Medfield, Mass.: Medfield Foundation, 1973. (b) (Mimeo.)

Spiegel, H. Hypnosis and transference. *Archives of General Psychiatry*, 1959, 1, 634-639.

Stankler, L. A critical assessment of the cure of warts by suggestion. *Practitioner*, 1967, 198, 690-694.

Staples, E.A., and Wilensky, H. A controlled Rorschach investigation of hypnotic age regression. *Journal of Projective Techniques and Personality Assessment*, 1968, 32, 246-252.

Starr, F.H., and Tobin, J.P. The effects of expectancy and hypnotic induction procedure on suggestibility. *American Journal of Clinical Hypnosis*, 1970, 12, 261-267.

Stoyva, J. The effect of suggested dreams on the length of rapid eye movement periods. Doctoral dissertation, University of Chicago, 1961.

Sulzberger, M.B., and Wolf, J. The treatment of warts by suggestion. *Medical Record*, 1934, 140, 552-557.

Surman, O.S., Gottlieb, S.K., Hackett, T.P., and Silverberg, E.L. Hypnosis in the treatment of warts. *Archives of General Psychiatry*. 1973, 28, 439-441.

Sutcliffe, J.P. "Credulous" and "sceptical" views of hypnotic phenomena: A review of certain evidence and methodology. *International Journal of Clinical and Experimental Hypnosis*, 1960, 8, 73-101.

Sutcliffe, J.P. "Credulous" and "skeptical" views of hypnotic phenomena: Experiments in esthesia, hallucination, and delusion. *Journal of Abnormal and Social Psychology*, 1961, 62, 189-200.

Tart, C.T. Effects of posthypnotic suggestion on the process of dreaming. Doctoral dissertation, University of North Carolina, 1963.

Tart, C.T. A comparison of suggested dreams occurring in hypnosis and sleep. *International Journal of Clinical and Experimental Hypnosis*, 1964, 12, 263-289.

Tart, C.T. Waking from sleep at a preselected time. *Journal of the American Society of Psychosomatic Dentistry and Medicine*, 1970, 17, 3-16.

Tart, C.T., and Dick, L. Conscious control of dreaming: I. The posthypnotic dream. *Journal of Abnormal Psychology*, 1970, 76, 304-315.

Tart, C.T., and Hilgard, E.R. Responsiveness to suggestions under "hypnosis" and "waking-imagination" conditions, a methodological observation. *International Journal of Clinical and Experimental Hypnosis*, 1966, 14, 247-256.

Taugher, V.J. Hypno-anesthesia. *Wisconsin Medical Journal*, 1958, 57, 95-96.

Taylor, A. The differentiation between simulated and true hypnotic regression by figure drawings. Masters thesis, College of the City of New York, 1950.

Tellegen, A., and Atkinson, G.A. "Fluidity," a trait independent of neuroticism and introversion, and related to hypnotic susceptibility. Department of Psychology, University of Minnesota, 1972.

Tenzel, J.H., and Taylor, R.L. An evaluation of hypnosis and suggestion as treatment for warts. *Psychosomatics*, 1969, 10, 252-257.

Thorne, D.E. Memory as related to hypnotic suggestion, procedure, and susceptibility. Doctoral dissertation, University of Utah, 1967.

Thorne, D.E. Amnesia and hypnosis. *International Journal of Clinical and Experimental Hypnosis*, 1969, 17, 225-241.

Thorne, D.E., and Hall, H.V. Hypnosis and amnesia revisited. Paper presented at the annual meeting of the Society for Clinical and Experimental Hypnosis, Palo Alto, 1969.

Timney, B.N., and Barber, T.X. Hypnotic induction and oral temperature. *International Journal of Clinical and Experimental Hypnosis*, 1969, 17, 121-132.

Tkach, W. A firsthand report from China: "I have seen acupuncture'work," says Nixon's doctor. *Today's Health*, 1972, 50, No. 7, 50-56.

Tracy, D.F. *Hypnosis*. New York: Sterling Publishing Co., 1952.

Troffer, S.A.H. Hypnotic age regression and cognitive functioning. Doctoral dissertation, Stanford University, 1966.

True, R.M. Experimental control in hypnotic age regression states. *Science*, 1949, 110, 583-584.

Tuckey, C.L. Psychotherapeutics; or treatment by hypnotism. *Woods Medical and Surgical Monographs*, 1889, 3, 721-795.

Ullman, M., and Dudek, S.Z. On the psyche and warts: II. Hypnotic suggestion and warts. *Psychosomatic Medicine*, 1960, 22, 68-76.

Unestahl, L.E. Hypnosis and hypnotic susceptibility. *Scandinavian Journal of Clinical and Experimental Hypnosis*, November 1969, 2.

Van Dyke, P.B. Hypnosis in surgery. *Journal of Abdominal Surgery*, 1965, 7, 1-5, 26-29.

Veith, I. Acupuncture: Ancient enigma to East and West. *American Journal of Psychiatry*, 1972, 129, 333-336.

Vollmer, H. Treatment of warts by suggestion. *Psychosomatic Medicine*, 1946, 8, 138-142.

Wall, P. An eye on the needle. *New Scientist*, July 20, 1972, 129-131.

Wallace, G., and Coppolino, C.A. Hypnosis in anesthesiology. *New York Journal of Medicine*, 1960, 60, 3258-3273.

Warren, F.D. Panel discussion: Acupuncture. In *Transcript of the Acupuncture Symposium*. Los Altos, Calif.: Academy of Parapsychology and Medicine, 1972. Pp. 86-92.

Watkins, J.G. *Hypnotherapy of War Neuroses*. New York: Ronald Press, 1949.

Watkins, J.G. Symposium on posthypnotic amnesia: Discussion. *International Journal of Clinical and Experimental Hypnosis*, 1966, 14, 139-149.

Webb, E.J., Campbell, D.T., Schwartz, R.D., and Sechrest, L. *Unobtrusive Measures: Nonreactive Research in the Social Sciences*. Chicago: Rand McNally, 1966.

Weinberg, N.H., and Zaslove, M. "Resistance" to systematic desensitization of phobias. *Journal of Clinical Psychology*, 1963, 14, 179-181.

Weitzenhoffer, A.M. *General Techniques of Hypnotism*. New York: Grune & Stratton, 1957.

Weitzenhoffer, A.M., and Hilgard, E.R. *Stanford Hypnotic Susceptibility Scale: Forms A and B*. Palo Alto, Calif.: Consulting Psychologists Press, 1959.

Weitzenhoffer, A.M., and Hilgard, E.R. *Stanford Hypnotic Susceptibility Scale: Form C*. Palo Alto, Calif.: Consulting Psychologists Press, 1962.

Weitzenhoffer, A.M., and Weitzenhoffer, G.B. Sex, transference, and susceptibility to hypnosis. *American Journal of Clinical Hypnosis*, 1958, 1, 15-24.

Weitzman, B. Behavior therapy and psychotherapy. *Psychological Review*, 1967, 74, 300-317.

Wells, W.R. Experiments in waking hypnosis for instructional purposes. *Journal of Abnormal and Social Psychology*, 1924, 18, 389-404.

Wenger, M.A., and Bagchi, B.K. Studies of autonomic functions in practitioners of Yoga in India. *Behavioral Science*, 1961, 6, 312-323.

Werbel, E.W. *One Surgeon's Experience with Hypnosis*. New York: Pageant Press, 1965.

Werbel, E.W. Hypnosis in serious surgical problems. *American Journal of Clinical Hypnosis*, 1967, 10, 44-47.

White, R.W. A preface to the theory of hypnotism. *Journal of Abnormal and Social Psychology*, 1941, 36, 477-505.

Williams, G.W. Difficulty in dehypnotizing. *Journal of Clinical and Experimental Hypnosis*, 1953, 1, 3-12.

Wilson, D.L. The role of confirmation of expectancies in hypnotic induction. Doctoral dissertation, University of North Carolina, 1967.

Wolberg, L.R. *Medical Hypnosis*. Vol. 1: *Principles of Hypnotherapy*. New York: Grune & Stratton, 1948.

Wolberg, L.R. *Hypnosis: Is It for You?* New York: Harcourt Brace Jovanovich, 1972.

Wolf, S., and Wolff, H.G. *Human Gastric Function: An Experimental Study of a Man and his Stomach*. (2nd Ed.) New York: Oxford University Press, 1947.

Wolff, L.V. The response to plantar stimulation in infancy. *American Journal Diseases of Childhood*, 1930, 39, 1176-1185.

Wolffenbüttel, E. Hypnosis and acupuncture, XIII: Summary and comments. *Revista Brasileira de Medicina*. 1968, 25, 827-831.

Wolpe, J. *Psychotherapy by Reciprocal Inhibition* Stanford: Stanford University Press, 1958.

Wolpe, J. *The Practice of Behavior Therapy*. New York: Pergamon Press, 1969.

Yates, A.J. Simulation and hypnotic age regression. *International Journal of Clinical and Experimental Hypnosis*, 1960, 8, 243-249.

Young, P.C. Hypnotic regression—fact or artifact? *Journal of Abnormal and Social Psychology*, 1940, 35, 273-278.

Zimbardo, P.G., Maslach, C., and Marshall, G. Hypnosis and the psychology of cognitive and behavioral control. Department of Psychology, Stanford University, 1970. (Mimeo.)

Name Index

Subject Index